Andrea Ciarrocchi
The Vermiform Appendix

Andrea Ciarrocchi

The Vermiform Appendix

—

DE GRUYTER

Author
Dr. Andrea Ciarrocchi
General and Emergency Surgery
ASL Teramo
Circonvallazione Ragusa, 1
64100 Teramo
Italy
ciarro85@hotmail.it

ISBN 978-3-11-914341-7
e-ISBN (PDF) 978-3-11-221978-2
e-ISBN (EPUB) 978-3-11-222002-3

Library of Congress Control Number: 2025940761

Bibliographic information published by the Deutsche Nationalbibliothek
The Deutsche Nationalbibliothek lists this publication in the Deutsche Nationalbibliografie;
detailed bibliographic data are available on the internet at http://dnb.dnb.de.

www.degruyter.com
Questions about General Product Safety Regulation:
productsafety@degruyterbrill.com

Preface

This book arises from the need to provide a comprehensive and up-to-date overview of an often-overlooked organ—the vermiform appendix—whose anatomical, physiological, and pathological complexity deserves in-depth exploration. The goal is to bridge the gap between traditional knowledge and recent scientific discoveries, adopting a multidisciplinary approach that spans embryology, surgery, inflammatory diseases, and malignancies.

The text is structured into three main chapters. The first, "Embryology, anatomy, and physiology", explores the structural and functional foundations of the appendix, including its frequently underestimated immunological role. The second, "Inflammatory diseases", focuses on diagnosis, techniques, and challenges in special populations. The third, "Malignancies", examines both primary and metastatic cancers through diagnostic criteria and treatment options.

Each section integrates clinical evidence and treatment options. The language is deliberately clear to make complex concepts accessible to students, physicians, and researchers without compromising scientific rigor.

I extend my deepest gratitude to the colleagues and mentors who provided constructive feedback, as well as the patients whose stories inspired this work. A special acknowledgment goes to my family for their unwavering support during the writing process.

I hope this book serves as both a practical resource and a catalyst for further research into an organ that, despite its small size, still holds many mysteries.

https://doi.org/10.1515/9783112219782-202

Contents

Chapter 1
Embryology, anatomy, and physiology

1.1 Introduction

The appendix is a small outpouching of the colon, located at the distal end of the cecum. It is a slender, tube-like structure with a blind end. The term "vermiform appendix" originates from Latin and translates to "worm-like appearance." This structure was first described by Berengario da Carpi in 1521, although Leonardo da Vinci had already depicted it in his anatomical drawings in 1492. The term "vermiform appendix" was later coined by Vido Vidius (Guido Guidi) in 1530.

The appendix is present in all hominids, including apes and humans. Additionally, several other mammals, such as rabbits and wombats, possess a cecal appendage similar to the human appendix. For a long time, its function remained unknown, leading to its classification as a vestigial organ with no apparent role. It was once believed that the human appendix would gradually diminish or disappear over the course of evolution. Charles Darwin and other proponents of evolutionary theory identified the vermiform appendix as a rudimentary organ, considering its vestigial nature as evidence of human evolutionary history.

However, in recent years, growing scientific evidence has challenged this notion. Today, the appendix is recognized as playing an active role in the immune system, contributing to the body's defense against various pathogens.

1.2 Embryology

The understanding of the embryology of the vermiform appendix has evolved significantly over time, shaped by advances in anatomical studies, imaging techniques, molecular biology, and embryological research. Early anatomists had only a rudimentary understanding of its formation and function, viewing it primarily as a diverticulum of the cecum, but its embryological development remained largely speculative. Throughout the seventeenth and eighteenth centuries, anatomical dissections became more frequent, allowing scientists to describe the appendix's structure with greater accuracy, yet it was still considered a vestigial remnant. The nineteenth century saw further advancements, with figures like Henry Gray providing detailed anatomical descriptions, though histological and embryological studies were still in their infancy. It wasn't until the late nineteenth and early twentieth centuries that the appendix was recognized as an outgrowth of the cecum during early fetal development, appearing as a bud around the 6th week of gestation. Researchers noted that the appendix and cecum formed from the caudal limb of the midgut loop, which underwent rotation and migration to its final position, and they began to document its delayed growth

https://doi.org/10.1515/9783112219782-001

compared to the rest of the cecum. The identification of lymphoid tissue within the appendix led to early speculations about its immune function rather than it being purely vestigial. The mid-twentieth century saw significant progress due to advances in histological techniques, electron microscopy, and immunohistochemistry, leading to key discoveries such as the confirmation that lymphatic tissue appears in the appendix around the 14th week of gestation, with lymphoid nodules forming between the fourth and fifth months, supporting the hypothesis of its immune function. Studies also revealed that the appendix's position is highly variable during fetal development, ranging from subcecal to postileal or pelvic locations, depending on the ongoing growth and rotation of the intestines. Additionally, research highlighted the role of mesenteric development in stabilizing the appendix's final positioning by the end of gestation. By the late twentieth century, the appendix was no longer universally considered vestigial, and its embryological complexity was increasingly recognized. The twenty-first century has brought even greater insights through genetic and evolutionary research, with advanced imaging techniques such as high-resolution ultrasound and MRI allowing for precise visualization of fetal gut development. Genetic studies have identified several genes involved in gut morphogenesis, suggesting that appendix formation is a regulated developmental process rather than a random evolutionary remnant. Comparative embryology has shown that many mammals, including rabbits, wombats, and some primates, possess cecal appendages similar to the human appendix, suggesting that this structure has evolved multiple times in different species, likely as an adaptation for immune function and gut microbiota regulation. The discovery that the appendix serves as a reservoir for beneficial gut bacteria further reinforces its functional significance. Over the centuries, the embryology of the appendix has gone from being an anatomical curiosity to a well-studied developmental process with clinical and evolutionary importance, reflecting the broader advancements in embryology, genetics, and medical imaging. While further research is still needed to fully elucidate the genetic and molecular pathways governing appendiceal development, it is now clear that the appendix is more than a mere evolutionary remnant – it is an actively developing structure with important physiological roles.

The development of the vermiform appendix begins as part of the midgut, which arises from the primitive gut tube. The midgut is initially a straight tubular structure that is continuous with the foregut and hindgut. By the 4th week of gestation, rapid proliferation of endodermal and mesodermal layers leads to the formation of the primary intestinal loop, which is suspended from the dorsal abdominal wall by the dorsal mesentery. This loop is characterized by two limbs: the cranial limb, which will form most of the small intestine, and the caudal limb, which will give rise to parts of the large intestine, including the distal ileum, cecum, appendix, ascending colon, and a portion of the transverse colon.

As embryonic development progresses, the midgut loop undergoes significant elongation, outpacing the growth of the embryonic abdominal cavity. This differential growth results in a temporary physiological herniation of the midgut into the extra-embryonic coelom within the umbilical cord around the 5th week. During this phase, the cecal diverticulum begins to emerge as a small outpouching from the caudal limb of the midgut loop. This diverticulum represents the earliest identifiable structure that will later differentiate into the cecum and the vermiform appendix.

By the 6th week of gestation, a small bud emerges from the rudimentary cecum, marking the formation of the primitive appendix. Initially, this structure appears as a minor diverticulum, with little distinction from the developing cecum. At this stage, the superior mesenteric artery plays a crucial role in supplying blood to the embryonic gut, ensuring proper development. The various segments of the primitive gut grow at different rates, contributing to the distinct morphological features of the digestive system. Notably, the lower portion of the cecum develops at a slower rate compared to its upper counterpart. This differential growth pattern results in the gradual elongation and differentiation of the appendix as a separate anatomical entity. As the cecum continues to expand, the appendix is progressively displaced upward and medially, assuming its characteristic narrow, elongated form. The midgut loop begins its characteristic counterclockwise rotation around the axis of the superior mesenteric artery. This initial 90-degree rotation sets the stage for further repositioning and elongation of the intestines, which will ultimately influence the final placement of the appendix and other components of the gastrointestinal tract.

Between the 6th and the 14th week of gestation, the development of the cecum and appendix is closely tied to the continued elongation, rotation, and fixation of the midgut. Around the 6th week, the midgut, including the cecal diverticulum, is still herniated into the extraembryonic coelom due to the limited space within the abdominal cavity. As the midgut continues to grow, it undergoes a second 180-degree counterclockwise rotation around the axis of the superior mesenteric artery, bringing the cecum and its appendage into a more anterior position relative to the rest of the midgut structures.

By the 10th week of gestation, the abdominal cavity has expanded sufficiently to accommodate the growing intestines, allowing for their return from the physiological umbilical herniation. As the midgut retracts into the abdomen, the cecum is initially positioned near the right upper quadrant, close to the liver. However, as fetal growth progresses, differential elongation of the ascending colon and modifications in the mesentery drive the cecum downward. During this period, the mesentery plays a crucial role in determining the final anatomical arrangement of the intestines. Initially, the cecum and appendix possess a mesentery that extends from the dorsal abdominal wall, but as the intestines rotate and settle into their final positions, portions of the mesentery fuse with the posterior peritoneum, leading to the partial retroperitoneal fixation of the ascending colon while the appendix retains its mobility.

By the 12th to 14th week of gestation, the cecum has typically reached the lower right quadrant, although its exact location can vary due to individual differences in mesenteric development and midgut rotation. The appendix, which arises from the posteromedial aspect of the cecum, continues to elongate during this period. Its final positioning – whether retrocecal, pelvic, or subcecal – is largely dependent on the degree of rotation and fixation of the mesentery. The vascularization of the appendix, primarily through the appendicular artery, a branch of the ileocolic artery, is also well established by this stage, ensuring adequate blood supply for further growth and differentiation.

Fitzgerald et al. reported that during the fetal period, the cecum is initially positioned in the lower right quadrant of the abdomen before undergoing its characteristic descent into the right iliac fossa. The final positioning of the appendix, however, is influenced by the development of the mesentery – a vital tissue responsible for vascular supply, lymphatic drainage, and structural support of the intestines. The mesentery undergoes significant modifications throughout fetal development, guiding the positioning of the digestive organs. By the 14th week of gestation, lymphatic tissue begins to develop within the appendix, with lymphoid nodules appearing between the 4th and 5th months. These nodules continue to proliferate after birth, playing an increasingly important role in immune function, particularly during childhood and adolescence, when the appendix reaches its peak lymphoid activity.

Interestingly, the anatomical location of the appendix differs between fetal life and adulthood due to the dynamic nature of intestinal development. While in adults the appendix is most commonly found in a retrocecal or pelvic position, its location during fetal development is more variable. Studies have shown that in fetuses, the appendix may assume subcecal, retrocecal, or postileal positions, reflecting the ongoing growth and repositioning of the intestines. These variations are largely attributed to the random torsion and rotation of the developing gut, which occurs during midgut development. Unlike in adulthood, where the mesentery stabilizes the intestines in a fixed configuration, the fetal digestive system remains relatively mobile, allowing for positional changes throughout gestation. Notably, no specific genetic determinants have been identified in regulating the torsion and final positioning of the appendix, suggesting that its orientation results from a combination of mechanical forces and developmental chance rather than programmed genetic instruction.

According to Kim et al., the superior or inferior extension of the appendix during the migration phase does not appear to influence its final anatomical relationship with the terminal ileum in either fetuses or adults. However, certain positional variations have been observed, particularly in cases where the appendix assumes a retro-ileal location, leading to a coiled orientation behind the ileocecal junction. Their study suggests that the liver surface may play a guiding role in posterior migration, with the final ascent of the liver influencing the appendix's positioning in relation to the cecum and ileum. These findings highlight the complexity of appendiceal development and underscore the intricate interplay between embryological growth patterns and spatial constraints within the abdominal cavity.

Between the 14th week of gestation and delivery, the cecum and appendix continue to develop in response to the overall growth of the intestines and abdominal cavity. At the beginning of this period, the cecum remains relatively high in the lower right quadrant but progressively migrates downward as the ascending colon elongates and the abdominal cavity expands. This descent is facilitated by the remodeling of the mesentery, which undergoes further fusion to the posterior abdominal wall, fixing the ascending colon in place while allowing the appendix to retain its intraperitoneal mobility. The appendix itself, which initially formed as a small diverticulum from the cecal bud, continues to elongate, becoming a narrow, tubular structure that gradually assumes its final shape. Its position varies, influenced by the degree of rotation and the specific attachments of the mesoappendix, which contains the appendicular artery and lymphatic structures necessary for its vascular and immune function.

As the appendix lengthens, its histological layers become more distinct. The mucosa, submucosa, muscularis, and serosa are well established by the third trimester, and while the appendix does not play a functional role in digestion, its immune function begins to emerge as lymphoid tissue accumulates within the submucosa. Though not yet fully developed, this lymphoid tissue foreshadows the appendix's postnatal role in gut-associated immune responses. The vascular supply of the appendix remains stable, with the appendicular artery, a branch of the ileocolic artery, ensuring proper perfusion as the structure grows. Meanwhile, autonomic innervation integrates the appendix into the enteric nervous system, although its precise function in fetal life remains minimal.

By the final weeks of gestation, the cecum has usually reached its definitive position in the right iliac fossa, although minor variations can occur due to individual differences in rotation and mesenteric fixation. The appendix, depending on these factors, may adopt a retrocecal, pelvic, subcecal, or preileal/postileal orientation, with the retrocecal position being the most common postnatally. At birth, the appendix appears disproportionately long in relation to the cecum, a feature that will gradually change as the cecum expands and develops its characteristic sac-like shape. While the appendix remains histologically immature at birth, its postnatal development continues with the progressive accumulation of lymphoid tissue, reaching peak function during childhood when it plays a more defined role in the immune system.

1.3 Development abnormalities

Developmental anomalies of the appendix are rare, with most variations encountered during surgery relating to the position of its tip. This positioning is influenced by factors such as the degree of cecal descent and peritoneal fixation, cecal configuration, appendiceal length, presence of adhesions, and the individual's body habitus. More unusual anomalies, including complete absence, ectopia, and duplication of the appendix, are even less frequent.

1.3.1 Congenital agenesis and atresia

Congenital agenesis of the appendix, first described by Morgagni, is believed to result from an insufficient differential growth between the cecum and appendix during fetal development, making their distinction difficult. Other proposed mechanisms include intrauterine vascular accidents, autoamputation, and appendiceal atresia – the rarest of these conditions. Appendiceal atresia occurs when the organ forms but is obstructed at birth due to luminal occlusion, whereas true agenesis implies a complete failure of formation. Notably, appendiceal agenesis is more commonly diagnosed in adults than in children. Some researchers suggest that in certain cases, what appears to be agenesis may instead be a missed intracecal appendix, concealed within the cecal wall.

1.3.2 Horseshoe appendix

Among the described anatomical variations, a particularly rare anomaly is the horseshoe appendix, characterized by two separate points of attachment to the cecum, forming a loop. Only a handful of cases have been reported, and none have been diagnosed preoperatively. This suggests that some instances may go unrecognized in patients who do not undergo abdominal surgery or imaging. Some authors propose that an appendico-cecal fistula could contribute to the formation of a horseshoe appendix. Pathological examination may suggest a congenital origin due to the fistula's morphology and lack of inflammation, but its extreme rarity means that its precise etiology remains uncertain.

1.3.3 Appendiceal duplication

Appendiceal duplication is another rare anomaly, with an estimated incidence ranging from 0.004% to 0.009%. Most cases diagnosed in childhood present as surgical emergencies, often associated with other congenital anomalies affecting the gastrointestinal, genitourinary, and vertebral structures, leading to complex clinical presentations. In adults, appendiceal duplication is typically discovered incidentally during appendectomy for acute appendicitis.

Wallbridge classified appendiceal duplications into three types:
- Type A: a single appendiceal base with partial duplication along its length.
- Type B: two completely separate appendices:
  - B1 (bird-like variant): Symmetrically positioned on either side of the ileocecal valve.
  - B2 (taenia-colic variant): One normally positioned appendix and another, usually rudimentary, arising from the cecum along the taenia.
- Type C: A double cecum, each with its own appendix.

These variations pose significant diagnostic challenges. Type A duplication can resemble appendiceal diverticulosis, present in up to 2.1% of surgical specimens, whereas Type B2 duplication can be mistaken for solitary cecal diverticula, particularly when an inflamed diverticulum is near the ileocecal junction. Histological examination helps differentiate these entities, as true appendiceal structures contain lymphoid tissue within the mucosa.

A systematic review identified 141 documented cases of appendiceal duplication. According to Nageswaran et al., an anteriorly positioned appendix, especially if separated from the taenia convergence, or the presence of clinical or radiological signs of appendicitis with a normal appendix, should prompt careful exploration of the cecal pole and retrocecal space for possible duplication. The increasing reliance on laparoscopic surgery, which lacks tactile feedback, further underscores the importance of heightened awareness regarding these anomalies.

Various theories exist regarding the embryological basis of appendiceal duplication. Some authors suggest that B2 duplication arises from a persistent "transient appendix" that appears during the 6th and 7th weeks of gestation. B1 duplication is thought to result from incomplete cloacal differentiation, while Type C may stem from partial twinning of hindgut structures. Notably, Type B1 and Type C duplications are often associated with other congenital anomalies, particularly reproductive tract duplications and anorectal malformations.

1.3.4 Other appendiceal abnormalities

Additional appendiceal abnormalities include congenital diverticula and heterotopic mucosa, which may contain pancreatic, gastric, or esophageal tissue. Another rare variation involves an intracecal appendix, in which the appendix becomes incorporated into the cecal wall, making it difficult to visualize during surgery. This likely occurs during midgut rotation and fixation when the appendix is closely apposed to the cecum, eventually fusing with its wall. In such cases, the hallmark feature is the absence of the mesoappendix, as this structure is incorporated into the cecal tissue.

1.3.5 Ectopic appendices and appendiceal herniation

Ectopic appendices are exceptionally rare. Reports describe appendices located in the thorax, lumbar region, and even the gluteal area, usually in association with congenital anomalies such as diaphragmatic hernias or piriformis muscle agenesis. Another unique condition is the umbilical appendix, in which appendiceal tissue remains extra-abdominal due to a failure of intestinal loops to fully return during embryogenesis. If an umbilical appendix is unrecognized at birth, improper umbilical cord clamping can lead to the formation of an appendico-umbilical fistula, establishing a pathological connection between the intestine and the skin.

Amyand's hernia, characterized by the presence of the appendix within an inguinal hernia sac, is another rare finding. While typically asymptomatic, it can become complicated by incarceration, strangulation, or even perforation. Though most frequently found in inguinal and femoral hernias, incarcerated appendices have also been reported in umbilical and incisional hernias. Given its nonspecific presentation, Amyand's hernia poses a diagnostic challenge.

1.3.6 Surgical and diagnostic implications

With the increasing prevalence of laparoscopic surgery, the reduced tactile feedback during procedures makes it even more essential for surgeons to be aware of these rare anomalies, as their subtle presentations may otherwise go unnoticed. Surgeons performing appendectomies should remain vigilant for anatomical variations, particularly in cases of recurrent right lower quadrant pain following prior appendectomy, as this could indicate an undiagnosed duplication. Similarly, imaging specialists should consider rare appendiceal anomalies when interpreting CT or MRI scans of the cecal region.

Greater awareness of appendiceal anomalies can improve diagnostic accuracy, prevent misdiagnosis, and guide appropriate surgical management, ultimately leading to better patient outcomes.

1.4 Normal and comparative anatomy

Understanding the anatomy of the vermiform appendix, which varies among individuals, is essential for both diagnosing appendicitis and performing a successful appendectomy. Typically, the appendix is located in the lower right quadrant of the abdomen. However, it may also be found in the upper left quadrant, the left anterior paramidline, or along the lower midline. Less common locations result from developmental anomalies, which were discussed in the previous section.

The position of the appendix is largely influenced by the orientation of the cecum, which itself can vary due to factors such as intestinal malrotation, developmental anomalies, or post-surgical changes. The appendix most commonly adopts a retrocecal position, meaning it extends posteriorly behind the cecum, a variation observed in approximately 65% of cases. In this position, the appendix may be partially covered by the cecum, making it less accessible during clinical examinations and more challenging to visualize using ultrasonography. Retrocecal appendicitis often presents with atypical symptoms, including flank or back pain, rather than the classic periumbilical and right lower quadrant pain.

In about 30% of individuals, the appendix assumes a pelvic position, where it descends into the pelvis, sometimes lying adjacent to the rectum, bladder, or even the uterus in females. Pelvic appendicitis may cause symptoms that mimic gynecological or urinary conditions, such as dysuria, increased urinary frequency, or deep pelvic pain. In rare instances, the appendix can be located in a subcecal position, lying directly beneath the cecum, or in a pre-ileal or post-ileal position, where it is found anterior or posterior to the terminal ileum, respectively. These variations are less common but can influence the clinical presentation of appendicitis, leading to diagnostic challenges.

In cases of situs inversus totalis, a rare congenital condition in which visceral organs are mirrored from their normal positions, the appendix is found in the left lower quadrant, mirroring its usual placement on the right. Similarly, intestinal malrotation, a developmental anomaly affecting the rotation of the midgut during embryogenesis, can result in the appendix being positioned in unusual locations, including the upper abdomen. Such anatomical variations necessitate careful consideration during diagnostic imaging and surgical planning to avoid misdiagnosis or inadvertent injury to adjacent structures.

The appendix is usually attached to the posteromedial wall of the cecum, approximately two centimeters below the ileocecal valve. It lies anterior to the iliopsoas and lumbar plexus, and posterior to the greater omentum and anterior abdominal wall. Suspended from the terminal ileum by a triangular fold of mesentery known as the mesoappendix – which also connects it to the cecum – the appendix has an average length of 8–9 cm. While the base of the appendix may vary slightly in location, the distance between its base and the ileocecal valve remains relatively constant. This consistency can aid in localizing the appendix during surgical or imaging procedures, with studies reporting a mean distance of approximately 25.69 mm.

The lumen of the distal appendix is typically partially occluded, whereas its proximal end opens into the cecum about 2.5 cm below the ileocecal valve. At this junction, a mucosal fold known as the valve of Gerlach is present. Although the appendix's length is highly variable, its diameter remains relatively consistent, a fact supported by several computed tomography studies. Evolutionary pressures seem to have maintained a stable appendiceal diameter, while its length is subject to greater variability. Additionally, the thickness of the appendiceal wall is a critical diagnostic criterion for inflammation in imaging examinations.

Histologically, the appendiceal wall resembles that of the colon but contains a higher concentration of lymphoid follicles, which are prominent within the lamina propria and submucosa. These follicles are typically organized in a nodular pattern, with germinal centers actively producing B lymphocytes. The mucosal surface features dome-like elevations that correspond to the apical poles of these follicles, contributing to the unique immune function of the appendix. Surrounding these domes are openings of the crypts of Lieberkühn, which are arranged in circular and radial patterns and lined by a simple columnar epithelium interspersed with goblet cells, enteroendocrine cells, and Paneth cells. The latter, located at the base of the crypts, secrete antimicrobial peptides such as defensins and lysozyme, which help regulate the microbiota within the appendiceal lumen.

The appendix has an extensive lymphatic network, with large vessels draining from the periphery of the follicles. Lymphatic drainage proceeds through the muscularis externa into the sub-serosal plexus, from which it is collected via vessels in the mesoappendix and transported to regional lymph nodes, primarily the ileocecal nodes. The amount of lymphoid tissue in the appendix is not static; it peaks during early life, particularly in childhood and adolescence, when the appendix plays a significant role in the immune response. However, after the age of 30, progressive involution occurs, leading to a decline in lymphoid tissue and a gradual increase in fibrous replacement.

The appendiceal wall is composed of four distinct layers: the mucosa, submucosa, muscularis externa, and serosa. The mucosa is rich in lymphoid aggregates, which contribute to its immune surveillance role. The submucosa, in addition to containing dense lymphoid tissue, is also characterized by a loose connective tissue matrix that provides support to blood vessels and lymphatic channels. The muscularis externa consists of an inner circular and an outer longitudinal layer of smooth muscle, facilitating peristaltic movements that aid in the expulsion of luminal contents. Unlike in the colon, the longitudinal muscle layer is more uniformly distributed rather than being concentrated in taeniae coli.

Within the appendix, lymphocytes proliferate within a maturing mesenchymal framework composed of reticular connective tissue. Reticular cells extend long processes to maintain structural integrity, while collagenous connective tissue surrounds the lymphatic sinuses and extends between lymphoid follicles. The presence of macrophages and dendritic cells within the follicular regions highlights the appendix's role in antigen presentation and immune modulation. Additionally, the high density of plasma cells in the lamina propria supports the production of secretory immunoglobulin A (sIgA), which contributes to mucosal immunity by neutralizing pathogens and maintaining homeostasis in the gut microbiota.

The epithelium of the appendix also plays a role in immune interactions. M (microfold) cells, which are found overlying the lymphoid follicles, facilitate antigen sampling from the lumen and mediate communication between luminal microorganisms and immune cells. These cells lack microvilli but possess a specialized basal pocket that allows for direct interaction with dendritic cells and lymphocytes, promoting an adaptive immune response.

The appendix, while histologically resembling the colon, possesses unique structural and functional characteristics that support its role as an immunological organ. The interplay between lymphoid tissue, specialized epithelium, and an intricate vascular and lymphatic network underscores its function in maintaining gut homeostasis, particularly in early life.

The appendix receives its arterial blood supply from the appendicular artery, a slender but functionally critical branch that typically arises from the ileocolic artery. However, variations in its origin have been documented, with studies showing that the appendicular artery can also arise from the posterior cecal (13%), anterior cecal (4.25%), medial ileocolic (8.25%), or ileal arteries (4.25%). This variability in vascular anatomy is important in surgical planning, particularly during appendectomy, as unrecognized anomalous branches may lead to incomplete ligation and subsequent hemorrhage.

The appendicular artery follows a retrocecal or mesoappendicular course, running within the free edge of the mesoappendix, where it is closely associated with the appendicular vein and accompanying lymphatic vessels. It provides several small branches to the mesoappendix before penetrating the muscularis externa of the appendix to form an intramural capillary network that supplies the mucosa, submucosa, and muscular layers. Unlike other sections of the alimentary canal, which benefit from an extensive network of anastomosing vessels, the appendix is uniquely dependent on this single, terminal end-artery. This anatomical feature renders it particularly vulnerable to ischemic injury in the setting of acute infection, inflammation, or mechanical obstruction.

When appendicitis progresses, luminal obstruction – often caused by a fecalith, lymphoid hyperplasia, or neoplasm – leads to increased intraluminal pressure, which compresses the venous outflow while arterial inflow continues, resulting in vascular congestion. This congestion predisposes the appendicular wall to thrombosis of the end-artery, leading to ischemia and, ultimately, necrosis. The lack of significant collateral circulation means that once arterial perfusion is compromised, gangrene and perforation can rapidly follow, often within 24–48 h of symptom onset.

Venous drainage of the appendix occurs through the appendicular vein, which follows the course of the artery and empties into the cecal venous system before merging with the ileocolic vein. From there, venous blood drains into the superior mesenteric vein, which is a major tributary of the hepatic portal system. This venous drainage pattern has clinical significance, as it provides a direct pathway for septic emboli from an infected appendix to reach the liver, potentially leading to pyogenic liver abscesses. Cases of appendicitis complicated by septic thrombophlebitis of the portal venous system, known as pylephlebitis, highlight the importance of early recognition and treatment of appendiceal infections.

Lymphatic drainage of the appendix follows the course of the ileocolic artery, initially collecting within the mesoappendix before passing through a series of lymph nodes along the ileocolic vessels. These include the appendicular, ileocolic, and superior mesenteric lymph nodes, which play a key role in immune surveillance. The abundant lymphoid tissue within the appendix contributes to the early activation of immune responses in gastrointestinal infections, but it can also be a site of pathological obstruction, as seen in appendicitis secondary to reactive lymphoid hyperplasia.

Neural regulation of appendiceal function is mediated by both the autonomic and enteric nervous systems. The myenteric plexus of the appendix exhibits distinct neuronal networks compared to other parts of the intestine, contributing to its motility and secretory functions. Sympathetic innervation originates from the celiac and superior mesenteric ganglia, regulating vasomotor tone and reducing peristalsis during stress responses. Parasympathetic innervation is provided by the vagus nerve, which promotes secretomotor activity and maintains the baseline motility of the appendix.

Sensory afferents from the appendix travel via sympathetic pathways, with pain fibers entering the spinal cord at the T10 level. This explains the characteristic early visceral pain of appendicitis, which is typically perceived as diffuse discomfort around the periumbilical region. As inflammation progresses and involves the parietal peritoneum, somatic nerve fibers become engaged, leading to the more localized and sharper pain in the right lower quadrant known as McBurney's point tenderness. This transition from visceral to somatic pain is a hallmark of appendicitis and is essential in clinical diagnosis.

From a comparative anatomical perspective, defining an appendix requires clear morphological and functional criteria, as outlined by Fisher R. in her comprehensive review. Key characteristics include a narrow, blind-ending lumen, a distinct thick-walled apex, and a significant concentration of lymphoid tissue within the mucosa and submucosa. While the presence of a vermiform appendix is widely accepted in humans and hominoid apes, its identification in other species remains a topic of debate. Reider et al. proposed that appendage-like structures in lower primates may be transient, formed by peristaltic contractions of the apical cecal segment. This theory may explain the variable constriction seen across different species, particularly in taxa where the appendix appears inconsistently or is difficult to distinguish from the cecum. However, factors such as individual variation, preservation quality, and underlying pathology could also contribute to the observed anatomical differences. Additionally, age-related changes complicate comparative studies, as appendiceal shape and lymphoid tissue concentration fluctuate over time, with peak development typically occurring in early life and subsequent involution in adulthood.

A well-defined vermiform appendix is consistently found in hominoid apes, including gorillas, chimpanzees, orangutans, and gibbons. In these species, the appendix originates from the posteromedial cecal wall at the junction of the taeniae coli, similar to the human appendix. Compared to monkeys, humans exhibit an increased appendiceal diameter and a relative reduction in cecal length, suggesting an evolutionary trend toward a more specialized immunological function rather than a primary role in digestion. Some other mammals, such as wombats, certain rodents, and rabbits, also possess an appendix-like structure. Several primates exhibit both a cecum and an appendix or an intermediate structure rich in lymphoid tissue and bacterial activity, suggesting a homologous function to the human appendix. These structures may play a role in microbial fermentation and immune surveillance, particularly in species with a herbivorous or omnivorous diet.

In certain non-primate mammals, such as rabbits and prehensile-tailed porcupines, the appendix is morphologically distinct from the cecum, with a noticeable reduction in intestinal caliber at the junction between the two. Their appendices contain abundant lymphoid tissue, akin to the human appendix, and contribute to the maintenance of gut-associated lymphoid tissue (GALT). In these species, the appendix plays a role in regulating the intestinal microbiota and may serve as a site for bacterial recolonization following gastrointestinal infections. The presence of a distinct lymphoid-rich appendix in some species, but not others, raises questions regarding the evolutionary pressures shaping its retention or loss.

In hominoid apes, the appendix is characterized by thick apical walls and a dense concentration of lymphoid follicles, though wall thickness alone does not appear to correlate with appendiceal function. Studies suggest that lymphoid concentration alone is insufficient to define an appendix, as germinal centers are present even in taxa lacking true cecal diverticula. Furthermore, the specimen's age must be considered when comparing lymphoid tissue across species, as the prominence of lymphoid follicles declines with age in both humans and nonhuman primates. The current scarcity of high-quality anatomical and histological data limits definitive conclusions regarding the comparative anatomy of the appendix, particularly in species where cecal and appendiceal structures exhibit a continuum rather than a clear distinction.

Some species exhibit "appendix-like structures" despite lacking a true cecum. Such formations occur at the junction of the small and large intestines in extant monotremes, certain birds, and some actinopterygians (ray-finned fishes). In these cases, the structures are often associated with microbial fermentation, immune function, or both. Cladistic analyses suggest that the appendix has been lost multiple times throughout evolutionary history, an observation that aligns with its absence in some rodents and potentially certain primates. The selective pressures responsible for these evolutionary losses remain unclear but may relate to dietary shifts, gut microbiome adaptations, and social behaviors that mitigate the impact of intestinal pathogens on population health. In species with a high-fiber diet, for example, an enlarged cecum often serves a comparable function, housing cellulose-digesting bacteria and lymphoid tissue that collectively support digestion and immune function.

The appendix exhibits significant morphological variation across species, with hominoid primates and select non-primate mammals possessing well-defined structures analogous to the human appendix. While the primary function of the appendix has likely shifted from digestion to immune regulation over evolutionary time, its presence, absence, and degree of development in different taxa underscore the complex interplay of evolutionary pressures shaping its role within the gastrointestinal tract.

1.5 Appendix in veterinary medicine

In veterinary medicine, the appendix is largely considered a vestigial or functionally insignificant structure in most species, with notable differences compared to its role in humans. While humans and some primates possess a distinct vermiform appendix, many other mammals, including dogs, cats, and most carnivores, either lack an appendix entirely or have a structure that differs in both function and morphology. Instead of a well-defined appendix, these animals often have an enlarged cecum, which plays a critical role in digestion, particularly in species that rely on a plant-based diet. The cecum serves as a fermentation chamber where microbial populations aid in breaking down fibrous plant materials, facilitating the digestion of cellulose and other complex carbohydrates. This function is especially important in herbivorous and hindgut-fermenting species such as rabbits, rodents, horses, and some marsupials. In these animals, the cecum and its associated microbiota contribute significantly to overall gut health and nutrition by synthesizing vitamins, short-chain fatty acids, and other essential nutrients.

Although the appendix itself is not a major clinical concern in veterinary practice, conditions affecting the cecum can have significant implications for animal health. In species with a well-developed cecum, such as rabbits and guinea pigs, disorders such as typhlitis (inflammation of the cecum), cecal impaction, dysbiosis, and enteric infections can lead to severe gastrointestinal disturbances, weight loss, and even life-threatening conditions. Typhlitis in rabbits, for example, can be caused by bacterial infections, dietary imbalances, or antibiotic-induced disruption of the normal gut flora, leading to bloating, diarrhea, and systemic illness. In horses, cecal impaction is a serious condition that can result in colic, a common and sometimes fatal equine emergency. Treatment for these conditions often involves dietary management, antibiotics (used with caution to avoid further microbiota disruption), probiotics, fluid therapy, and, in severe cases, surgical intervention.

Comparatively, in carnivorous species such as dogs and cats, the cecum is relatively small and does not play a significant role in digestion. However, while appendicitis is almost nonexistent in these animals due to the absence of a distinct appendix, conditions such as cecal inversion, neoplasia, or secondary bacterial infections may still affect the region. In rare cases, foreign bodies or parasites can lead to cecal irritation, requiring medical or surgical intervention. In ruminants, including cattle, sheep, and goats, the cecum is part of a highly specialized digestive system that primarily relies on the fermentation process occurring in the forestomach. Disorders involving the cecum in these animals are uncommon but can include issues such as gas accumulation, cecal dilation, or volvulus, which may require veterinary intervention.

From an evolutionary perspective, the presence or absence of an appendix and its variations across species highlight the adaptability of gastrointestinal anatomy to different dietary and ecological niches. The appendix is believed to have evolved as a specialized immune organ, housing lymphoid tissue that supports gut-associated lymphoid function, particularly in species that rely on a microbiome-driven digestive system. This function is still present in some primates, where the appendix is thought to serve as a reservoir for beneficial bacteria that help repopulate the gut flora after infections or disruptions. While this theory is well-supported in human medicine, its relevance in veterinary medicine remains an area of ongoing research.

Overall, while the appendix itself is not a primary focus in veterinary medicine, understanding species-specific differences in gastrointestinal anatomy is crucial for diagnosing and managing conditions that affect related structures such as the cecum. Veterinarians must consider these anatomical and functional differences when evaluating digestive disorders, formulating treatment plans, and advising pet owners and livestock managers on proper dietary and medical care. In cases where surgical intervention is required, such as cecal impaction or volvulus, knowledge of comparative anatomy ensures that the correct approach is taken for each species. Further research into the evolutionary and immunological significance of the appendix in various animals may continue to provide insights into its residual functions and potential clinical relevance.

1.6 Acute appendicitis in animals

Acute appendicitis in animals is a relatively rare condition compared to its prevalence in humans, largely due to anatomical differences among species. While many mammals, including primates and some rodents, possess an appendix or a cecal diverticulum with immune functions, true appendicitis is uncommon outside of humans. In domestic animals such as dogs and cats, the appendix is either absent or functionally different, as their cecum plays a more significant role in digestion rather than harboring lymphoid tissue. However, in certain species such as rabbits, where the appendix is a well-developed, lymphoid-rich organ crucial for hindgut fermentation, inflammation of this structure can occur, albeit under different pathological circumstances than in humans. When appendicitis or cecal impaction does develop in animals, it is often secondary to bacterial infections, foreign body obstruction, or parasitic infestations. Clinical signs may include abdominal pain, lethargy, anorexia, and signs of gastrointestinal distress such as diarrhea or constipation. Diagnosis is challenging due to the nonspecific nature of symptoms and the difficulty in imaging the small organ in veterinary practice. In species where appendicitis is documented, such as nonhuman primates, treatment typically involves surgical removal of the inflamed appendix, supported by antibiotics and symptomatic care. Understanding appendicitis in animals is not only relevant for veterinary medicine but also provides comparative insights into the evolutionary and immunological significance of the appendix across different species.

1.7 The physiology of the safe house

Until recently, the appendix was considered a rudimentary organ with no real function, but modern research has revealed its crucial role in immune function and gut microbiota homeostasis. The appendix is now understood to act as a safe house for beneficial gut bacteria, particularly during and after episodes of diarrheal illness that can purge the intestinal microbiome. This role is closely tied to its substantial concentration of GALT, which allows it to serve as an immunological organ that interacts dynamically with the host's microbiota. The relationship between mammals and their gut bacteria is symbiotic, with microorganisms relying on the host for nutrients and habitat while in turn contributing to digestion, immune system development, and pathogen defense. If the appendix were merely a vestige of a larger ancestral cecum that had lost its digestive function, one would not expect to find both an appendix and an enlarged cecum in the same species, yet several mammals, including primates, rodents, and diprotodont marsupials, possess both structures. This suggests that the appendix has undergone evolutionary modification, transitioning from a digestive role in cellulose digestion, which was prominent in herbivorous ancestors, to an immunological and microbial regulatory role in modern humans. Despite the loss of cellulose digestion in the human cecum, the appendix still harbors a diverse microbial community within biofilms, highlighting its preserved function in microbial homeostasis.

One of the most significant aspects of the appendix's role in maintaining intestinal health is its association with biofilms, which are aggregates of bacteria embedded in a self-produced extracellular matrix. These biofilms provide a stable environment for commensal bacteria, enhancing bacterial survival and diversity while also fostering interactions between bacteria and bacteriophages, the viruses that infect bacteria. The ability of the appendix to sustain these bacterial communities suggests that it has evolved as an immunological organ that supports a bacterial-bacteriophage complex, ensuring a continuous inoculation of the intestines. Studies of biofilm formation in animal models further emphasize the importance of the proximal end of the large intestine in microbial maintenance, and the appendix, located at the terminal end of the cecum, is particularly well-suited for this role. Unlike other parts of the colon that are constantly exposed to fecal matter and peristaltic flow, the appendix is relatively isolated, minimizing pathogen exposure while preserving a stable microbial niche. This isolation becomes particularly advantageous during diarrheal illnesses, which can lead to a rapid depletion of gut microbiota. The appendix, by harboring a reservoir of commensal bacteria, can repopulate the gut following such disruptions, ensuring the restoration of microbial balance.

Compared to the microbiota of the rest of the gut, the appendix harbors a distinct microbial composition, with a higher proportion of Firmicutes, which dominate its bacterial community, and a relatively lower abundance of Bacteroidetes. The presence of diverse microbial phyla, including Firmicutes, Bacteroidetes, Actinobacteria, and Proteobacteria, supports the hypothesis that the appendix serves as a long-term reservoir for commensal bacteria. Interestingly, certain genera typically associated with the oral cavity, such as Fusobacterium, Gemella, and Parvimonas, have also been detected in the appendix, reinforcing the idea that the appendix plays a role in immune modulation by maintaining a diverse microbial cohort beneficial to host health. The biofilm in the appendix consists of two layers, an inner layer that directly adheres to the intestinal epithelium and is insoluble, preventing direct contact between pathogenic bacteria and epithelial cells, and an outer layer that contains a looser aggregation of bacteria capable of responding to environmental changes. This biofilm contributes to gut health by continuously shedding bacteria, either as individual planktonic cells, which can aid in pathogen exclusion, or as biofilm fragments, which facilitate recolonization of beneficial bacteria throughout the gut.

The shedding mechanism of the appendiceal biofilm is particularly important during diarrheal illness when the turnover of enterocytes accelerates, leading to increased biofilm shedding and temporary loss of gut microbiota. Because the appendix is anatomically positioned in such a way that it avoids direct exposure to the fecal stream, it remains relatively protected from diarrheal clearance, ensuring that its microbial reservoir is preserved even when the rest of the intestinal microbiota is depleted. Cytokine-mediated immune responses further support the appendix's role in gut health, as diarrheal pathogens have been shown to induce mucin gene expression, increasing mucus production in a possible attempt to reinforce the gut's protective barrier. This response, particularly mediated by tumor necrosis factor-alpha (TNF-α), may serve as a defense mechanism aimed at maintaining gut integrity during infections, though its precise function remains an area of ongoing research.

From an evolutionary perspective, the strategic placement of the appendix at the terminal end of the cecum appears to be an adaptive feature that enhances its ability to function as a microbial safe house. In populations where diarrheal diseases are prevalent due to poor sanitation and limited access to medical care, the ability to rapidly restore gut microbiota following infection would be highly advantageous for survival. This perspective aligns with epidemiological data showing that appendicitis is more common in industrialized nations, where improved sanitation and modern healthcare have reduced the selective pressure to maintain a functional appendix. Conversely, in developing regions where diarrheal diseases remain a leading cause of mortality, the appendix's role in microbiome restoration may be more crucial. Reports from UNICEF and the World Health Organization indicate that diarrheal illnesses account for roughly one-fifth of global childhood deaths, reinforcing the importance of gut microbiome stability in human health. While appendicitis is often viewed as a medical burden, its prevalence in Western populations may reflect an evolutionary trade-off rather than an inherent pathological condition, with the appendix's primary function becoming less essential as sanitation and healthcare improve. In contrast, in environments where recurrent gastrointestinal infections pose a significant threat, the ability of the appendix to serve as a microbial reservoir capable of reseeding the gut flora may provide a critical survival advantage.

Ultimately, the appendix, long dismissed as a vestigial organ, is now recognized as an integral component of gut microbiota regulation and immune function. Its role as a microbial safe house allows it to preserve beneficial bacteria and facilitate gut repopulation following microbial disruptions. The presence of biofilms, its strategic anatomical positioning, and its immunological interactions all support the hypothesis that the appendix plays a fundamental role in maintaining intestinal homeostasis. While its significance in industrialized societies remains debated, its contribution to survival in populations with high exposure to diarrheal diseases is increasingly acknowledged. Future research will likely provide further insights into the complex interactions between the appendix, the immune system, and the gut microbiome, shedding new light on its role in human health and disease.

Laurin et al. suggest that the emergence of appendicitis as a common condition is closely tied to industrialization and that prior to the late nineteenth century, selection pressure against the appendix due to appendicitis was likely minimal. The advent of modern surgical techniques quickly countered any potential evolutionary pressure by effectively preventing mortality from appendicitis, making it unlikely that natural selection would eliminate the appendix. In an era of advanced healthcare, sanitation, and nutrition, the removal of the appendix does not appear to have any significant detrimental consequences, further reinforcing the idea that its role is less critical in developed nations. The primary function of the appendix seems to be in environments where rapid gut microbiome restoration following diarrheal illness is essential, a scenario that has been largely mitigated in industrialized societies. Access to clean water, effective sewage systems, probiotic-enriched food, and rigorous food safety regulations has drastically reduced the incidence and impact of diarrheal diseases in these regions, preventing widespread loss of gut flora due to infection. Additionally, the presence of medical interventions, including antibiotics, intravenous fluids, and nutritional support, further diminishes the necessity for an organ specialized in microbiota replenishment. This suggests that while the appendix may still be vital for populations in underdeveloped areas, where diarrheal diseases remain a major health threat, its function has become largely redundant in wealthier nations.

Despite morphological changes throughout evolution, the cecal appendix appears to be an ancient structure that has maintained a symbiotic relationship with host bacteria across a wide range of species. The presence of microbial biofilms in the gut is not exclusive to humans but is a feature observed in multiple animal lineages, including earthworms, amphibians, and various mammals such as koalas and rodents. This widespread distribution suggests that the appendix has historically played an integral role in microbial-host interactions, reinforcing gut homeostasis and immune function. However, like other immune structures that evolved in response to ancient threats – such as the spleen's role in protection against malaria or the tonsils' function in combating airborne pathogens – the appendix may have been rendered obsolete by improvements in public health and hygiene. Factors associated with industrialization, including changes in diet, medical interventions, and controlled food and water supplies, have reshaped the ecological pressures on the human gastrointestinal system, reducing the selective advantage once conferred by an appendix capable of microbiome restoration. The increasing prevalence of appendicitis in modern societies may be a byproduct of these shifts, indicating that while the appendix was once beneficial, its function has become less relevant and, under specific circumstances, even deleterious.

The role of the appendix in immune defense extends beyond microbiome maintenance, as evidenced by its interactions with bacterial pathogens such as *Clostridium difficile*. Im et al. in 2011 demonstrated that the appendix plays a protective role against *C. difficile* infections by promoting the migration and maturation of B cells in response to toxin A, a key virulence factor of the pathogen. The activated B cells enhance the production of toxin A-specific immunoglobulins (Ig), IgG and IgA, which are then released into the bloodstream, bolstering systemic immunity against *C. difficile*. This suggests that, rather than being an entirely redundant organ, the appendix retains an immunological function that may still be relevant under certain pathological conditions. Given the rise of antibiotic-resistant infections and the increasing recognition of the gut microbiome's role in overall health, the appendix's immunological contributions may warrant further investigation, particularly in the context of recurrent infections or dysbiosis-related diseases. Whether the appendix will continue to persist in human populations or gradually become an evolutionary relic remains uncertain, but its complex relationship with the immune system and gut microbiota suggests that its significance has not been entirely erased by modern advancements.

1.8 Immunologic role of the appendix

Similar to the intestinal wall of the colon, the appendiceal wall consists of four distinct layers: the mucosa, submucosa, muscularis externa, and serosa. However, the cellular composition, function, and immunological role of the appendix differ significantly from those of the colon. Notably, the presence of lymphoid follicles in the submucosa and lamina propria is a defining feature of the appendiceal wall, making it an essential component of the GALT. The molecular biology of the appendiceal tissue has been extensively described by Kooij et al., and the following sections summarize its immunological significance.

1.8.1 Immune cell distribution in the appendiceal layers

All layers of the appendix contain a complex and unique abundance of immune cells. The mucosa is composed of columnar epithelium with enterocytes and goblet cells, a lamina propria, and a muscularis mucosae. The lamina propria is particularly rich in IgA- and IgG-producing plasma cells, often located in close proximity to macrophages. Intraepithelial lymphocytes (IELs) within the appendix predominantly consist of small CD8+ regulatory T cells (Tregs), similar to those found in the colonic epithelium. These Treg cells play a crucial role in maintaining peripheral tolerance by regulating inflammatory responses and preventing autoimmune diseases.

The follicle-associated epithelium, also known as the dome epithelium, is situated above the lymphoid follicles. This region contains an increased number of IELs compared to the rest of the appendiceal and colonic epithelium. In addition to Treg cells, it houses M cells and human leukocyte antigen D-related (HLA-DR)-bearing T and B cells. Some IELs display morphological similarities to follicular center cells, leading to the hypothesis that they may originate from these follicles. The appendix also contains crypts of Lieberkühn, akin to the colon, but uniquely features Paneth cells at the base of these crypts. These Paneth cells are primarily responsible for producing antimicrobial peptides, contributing to the appendix's role in mucosal immunity.

The submucosa, largely composed of connective tissue, is distinguished by numerous lymphoid follicles extending from the submucosa into the lamina propria. While these follicles are absent in a healthy colon, they resemble Peyer's patches found in the small intestine. The mantle zone of the lymphoid follicles, predominantly located near the lumen, contains densely packed B lymphocytes and a smaller population of T lymphocytes. The germinal center, situated further from the lumen, houses macrophages, centroblasts, and proliferating B cells. Monoclonal expansion of these cells forms the follicle, and centrocytes subsequently differentiate within the light zone in association with follicular dendritic cells. These dendritic cells activate centrocytes via antigen presentation, stimulating Ig production. Through CD40-CD40L interactions with T cells, centrocytes can differentiate into plasmablasts or memory B cells.

The mixed cell zone, found between the dome epithelium and lymphoid follicles, contains macrophages and both B and T lymphocytes. The basal region of the lymphoid follicles, referred to as the T-cell area, contains macrophages and T cells, with an eightfold higher concentration of CD4+ T cells than CD8+ T cells. Natural killer T lymphocytes within the appendix contribute to immune signaling by producing cytokines and chemokines upon activation, as evidenced by CD45R expression. The chemokine CCL21 likely facilitates the recruitment of B and T lymphocytes to the appendiceal lymphoid tissue and promotes the migration of activated dendritic cells to lymph nodes.

1.8.2 Unique lymphocyte surface markers and immunological functions

Beyond differences in immune cell composition, appendiceal lymphocytes exhibit distinct surface molecule expression profiles compared to intestinal lymphocytes. In the lamina propria, the integrin subunit β7 is expressed at higher levels in T cells than in

T and B cells elsewhere in the intestine. Integrin α4β7 is primarily present on T cells in the lamina propria and epithelium, while integrin αEβ7 is mainly expressed on mucosal CD8+ T cells and dendritic cells. The interaction of α4β7 with mucosal addressin cell adhesion molecule 1 mediates lymphocyte recruitment via "tethering and rolling". Conversely, αEβ7 facilitates lymphocyte retention through its binding to E-cadherin. Intestinal dendritic cells expressing αEβ7 likely promote the differentiation of fork-head box protein 3-expressing Treg cells in response to bacterial antigens. A suppression of this differentiation could potentially lead to proinflammatory states.

CD5+ B lymphocytes, also known as B1 cells, are found in greater numbers in the appendix than in other parts of the gut, and their numbers increase during inflammation. These B1 cells produce IgM antibodies targeting a broad range of pathogens, initially independent of antigen presentation by T cells. This innate-like immune response mirrors that of intraepithelial lymphocytes. Their expansion during inflammation may be linked to microbiome shifts associated with acute appendicitis. Additionally, CD5+ B cells produce both anti-self antibodies and the anti-inflammatory cytokine IL-10, implicating them in autoimmune regulation.

sIgA and mucin contribute to biofilm formation by promoting bacterial agglutination and adhesion to the mucus layer. The appendix has a high density of mucin and sIgA-producing B cells in the mucosa, fostering a promicrobiotic environment that supports its role as a bacterial safe house. This function underlies its potential immunoregulatory influence on gut microbiota and inflammatory diseases.

1.8.3 The appendix and ulcerative colitis: a hypothetical link

The appendix has been implicated in the pathogenesis of ulcerative colitis (UC), although the exact mechanisms remain uncertain. Traditionally considered a vestigial organ, emerging evidence suggests that the appendix plays an active role in gut immunity, potentially influencing the onset and progression of UC. One prominent theory proposes that the appendix serves as a reservoir for beneficial microbiota, contributing to microbial homeostasis and shaping immune responses in the colon. In this model, the appendix helps repopulate the gut with commensal bacteria following disturbances, such as infections or antibiotic treatments. Its removal, therefore, may impair the ability of the gut to maintain microbial diversity, possibly exacerbating dysbiosis – a key factor in the pathogenesis of UC. Conversely, some researchers argue that in the context of UC, the appendix may instead harbor pro-inflammatory microbial communities, fueling chronic inflammation.

Another hypothesis suggests that the appendix actively participates in immunomodulation through cytokine production. Given its abundant lymphoid tissue, the appendix produces various immune mediators, including interleukins TNF-α, which may contribute to an inflammatory cascade extending to the colon and rectum. In this scenario, appendectomy could mitigate inflammation by reducing the source of pro-inflammatory signaling, leading to clinical improvement in some UC patients. Furthermore, the appendix is a major site of sIgA production, a key player in mucosal immunity. Its removal might stimulate GALT to compensate, leading to alterations in the IgA:IgG ratio in the colon. This shift in antibody-mediated immunity could impact disease severity and response to treatment.

Epidemiological studies examining the relationship between appendectomy and UC have produced conflicting results. Several large-scale population studies have reported that patients who underwent appendectomy – particularly before the age of 20 – exhibit a lower incidence of UC, later disease onset, reduced need for immunosuppressive therapy, and lower colectomy rates. These findings suggest a potential protective effect of appendectomy against UC development, possibly by removing a source of pro-inflammatory immune stimulation in genetically predisposed individuals. However, other studies have not consistently confirmed this association, and some have raised concerns about confounding factors, such as differences in immune status, genetic predisposition, or lifestyle influences.

In patients with established UC, therapeutic appendectomy has shown mixed results. Some retrospective and prospective studies suggest that appendectomy can lead to symptomatic improvement, particularly in individuals with ulcerative proctitis, a localized form of UC affecting the rectum. This benefit may arise from disrupting immune cross-talk between the appendix and the distal colon, thereby dampening inflammation. However, other studies have found no significant clinical impact, suggesting that the therapeutic effect of appendectomy may depend on multiple factors, including disease extent, duration, and the presence of appendiceal inflammation.

Recent prospective trials have provided further insights, indicating that appendectomy may significantly improve symptoms in a subset of UC patients, particularly those with mild to moderate disease or with proctitis-predominant involvement. Some mechanistic studies suggest that inflammation of the appendix, often referred to as "appendiceal UC" or "skip appendicitis," may be an early marker of disease activity, potentially playing a role in disease progression. This raises the possibility that appendectomy might be most effective in a specific disease phenotype rather than as a general treatment for UC.

Despite these findings, the role of appendectomy in UC remains an area of debate, highlighting the need for further research to clarify its immunological and microbial implications. Future studies, particularly those integrating microbiome analysis and immunological profiling, may help determine whether the appendix is primarily a protective or pathogenic organ in the context of UC. Additionally, identifying patient subgroups that are most likely to benefit from appendectomy could pave the way for more personalized approaches to managing UC, potentially reducing the need for long-term immunosuppressive therapy or colectomy in select cases.

1.8.4 The hygiene hypothesis and immune dysregulation

The hygiene hypothesis, later refined as the "biome depletion theory of immune disorders," proposes that reduced exposure to environmental microbes in industrialized societies leads to immune hyper-reactivity and an increased incidence of autoimmune and inflammatory diseases. This theory suggests that as modern sanitation, antibiotic use, and dietary changes have drastically altered the human microbiome, the immune system is deprived of the diverse microbial stimuli that helped shape its regulatory mechanisms over evolutionary history. Without these early-life microbial exposures, immune tolerance may be impaired, leading to an exaggerated inflammatory response to otherwise benign antigens.

The appendix, with its extensive lymphoid tissue, is thought to play a crucial role in immune system modulation, particularly in maintaining a healthy gut microbiota. It serves as a reservoir for commensal bacteria, facilitating microbial repopulation of the intestine following infections or disruptions caused by antibiotics. This function may be especially relevant in societies where microbial diversity has been compromised due to modern hygienic practices. When deprived of proper microbial stimulation, the appendix and its associated GALT may contribute to aberrant immune responses, increasing the risk of immune dysregulation.

Studies have demonstrated that helminth colonization – a common feature of pre-industrial human environments – can downregulate immune activity, alleviating symptoms of various immune-mediated conditions such as inflammatory bowel disease (IBD), allergies, and even multiple sclerosis. This aligns with the broader concept that an incompatibility between human biology and post-industrial lifestyles contributes to immune dysfunction. For instance, appendicitis and UC have been linked to dysbiosis, or an imbalance in gut microbiota, reinforcing the idea that microbial depletion may disrupt immune homeostasis in ways that promote inflammatory pathologies.

Beyond its role as a bacterial reservoir, the appendix acts as an integral part of the mucosal immune system, participating in antigen sampling and the education of immune cells. The presence of abundant lymphoid follicles suggests that the appendix may help regulate the gut's response to pathogens while simultaneously fostering immune tolerance to commensal microbes. This delicate balance is critical for gut homeostasis, as disruptions in immune regulation can lead to excessive inflammation, as seen in IBD and other autoimmune conditions.

While the appendix was historically considered a vestigial organ with little functional significance, emerging research continues to highlight its involvement in immune modulation and gut microbial ecology. Its role in inflammatory disease pathogenesis is an area of active investigation, with growing evidence suggesting that the appendix may act as a key player in immune regulation, particularly in the context of modern environmental and lifestyle changes. Understanding these interactions could pave the way for novel therapeutic approaches aimed at restoring immune balance and preventing immune-mediated diseases.

1.9 Future perspectives

Future research on the appendix is poised to uncover deeper insights into its immunological functions, evolutionary significance, and potential clinical applications. Historically considered a vestigial organ, recent studies have highlighted its role as a reservoir for beneficial gut microbiota and its involvement in mucosal immunity, particularly through its dense concentration of lymphoid tissue. Advances in microbiome research may further elucidate how the appendix contributes to gut homeostasis and resilience against infections such as *Clostridioides difficile*. Moreover, its potential role in immune system modulation raises intriguing questions about its influence on autoimmune and inflammatory diseases, including Crohn's disease and UC. Another promising avenue is regenerative medicine – understanding the appendix's cellular composition and immune activity could inspire novel therapeutic strategies for gastrointestinal and immune-related disorders. From an evolutionary perspective, comparative studies across species could provide insights into why the appendix persists in some lineages while being absent in others, shedding light on its adaptive advantages. Additionally, advancements in imaging, artificial intelligence (AI), and computational biology may refine the ability to predict and diagnose appendiceal diseases with greater accuracy, improving patient outcomes. Finally, as minimally invasive surgical techniques continue to evolve, research into appendiceal preservation versus routine removal in certain cases – such as incidental appendectomy – may redefine clinical guidelines, balancing the risks and benefits of maintaining this enigmatic organ.

The appendix's rich lymphoid tissue and its role in gut microbiome homeostasis have sparked interest in its potential applications in regenerative medicine. As a site of immune cell proliferation and interaction, the appendix could serve as a model for developing treatments for gastrointestinal and immune disorders. One promising avenue is leveraging its ability to harbor beneficial bacteria to support microbiome restoration therapies, particularly for patients suffering from recurrent infections like *C. difficile* or dysbiosis-related conditions. Additionally, the appendix's involvement in mucosal immunity suggests it may have regenerative potential in IBDs, such as Crohn's disease and UC, where targeted therapies could enhance its protective functions. Advances in tissue engineering may even allow for the development of bioengineered lymphoid structures inspired by the appendix, potentially aiding in immune system modulation and personalized medicine approaches. Furthermore, understanding appendiceal stem cell populations could open new possibilities for gut tissue regeneration, particularly in patients with severe intestinal damage. Future research into the appendix's immunological properties and cellular composition could thus lead to novel regenerative strategies, transforming our approach to both gastrointestinal and systemic diseases.

The concept of an artificial or bioengineered appendix is an emerging frontier in regenerative medicine, with potential applications in restoring gut homeostasis, immune function, and microbiome balance. Given the appendix's role as a reservoir for beneficial bacteria and its dense concentration of GALT, bioengineering an artificial appendix could provide therapeutic benefits for patients who have undergone appendectomy or suffer from microbiome-related disorders. Using advances in tissue engineering, scientists could develop a biocompatible scaffold seeded with patient-derived stem cells to recreate the structural and immunological functions of the appendix. This bioengineered organ could be designed to support microbial recolonization after disruptions caused by antibiotics, infections, or IBDs. Additionally, 3D bioprinting technologies may allow for the precise replication of the appendix's complex architecture, ensuring proper interaction with the surrounding gut environment. Another promising approach involves implantable probiotic reservoirs, mimicking the appendix's function as a microbial sanctuary, which could be particularly useful in treating recurrent *C. difficile* infections or post-antibiotic dysbiosis. Research into immunomodulatory therapies might also leverage the appendix's ability to support immune cell development, paving the way for artificial lymphoid structures capable of aiding in immune regulation. While still in early stages, the prospect of a bioengineered appendix represents a paradigm shift in personalized medicine, offering new solutions for gastrointestinal health and immune system modulation.

1.10 Artificial intelligence diagnostics

AI is transforming medical diagnostics by improving accuracy, efficiency, and accessibility through advanced machine learning, deep learning, and natural language processing algorithms. AI-driven tools are revolutionizing medical imaging, where convolutional neural networks analyze radiological scans, such as X-rays, MRIs, and CT scans, to detect early signs of diseases like cancer, stroke, and cardiovascular conditions, often matching or exceeding human performance. In laboratory medicine, AI enhances pathology and microbiology by identifying cancerous cells in biopsy slides, detecting hematologic disorders in blood smears, and predicting antimicrobial resistance patterns to optimize treatment strategies. Genomic medicine also benefits from AI, with deep learning models analyzing vast genetic datasets to detect mutations associated with hereditary diseases and cancers, thereby advancing precision medicine. Beyond diagnostics, AI plays a crucial role in predictive analytics, assessing electronic health records, wearable device data, and lifestyle factors to foresee disease risks, enabling early interventions for conditions like diabetes and sepsis. Natural language processing further expands AI's capabilities by analyzing unstructured clinical notes, extracting diagnostic insights, and supporting clinical decision-making. However, challenges remain, including biases in training datasets, the need for explainability in deep learning models, regulatory hurdles, and concerns over patient privacy and ethical AI implementation. Future advancements in AI diagnostics may involve multimodal AI systems integrating imaging, genomics, and real-time patient data, along with federated learning models that ensure privacy while improving diagnostic accuracy across multiple healthcare institutions. As AI-driven robotics and real-time decision-support systems continue to develop, their successful integration into clinical practice will depend on balancing technological innovation with ethical considerations, regulatory compliance, and effective collaboration between AI and human clinicians.

References

- Takabatake K, I.J. FH. A case of a horseshoe appendix. Surg Case Rep. 2016; 2: 140.
- Fuijkschot J, W.R. G, GP D, SV R, P.N. A neonate with an intact congenital umbilical appendix: An alternative theory on the etiology of the appendico-umbilical fistula. Pediatr Surg Int. 2006; 8: 689–93.
- al Hm. A tale of two appendices – An unexpected finding. J Surg Case Rep. 2012; 212: 5.
- Mahmood A, M.N. W, J.L. Acute abdominal pain presenting as a rare appendiceal duplication: A case report. J Med Case Rep. 2012; 8: 6.
- Barker DJ, M.J. Acute appendicitis, bathrooms, and diet in Britain and Ireland. Brit Med J Clin Res Ed. 1988; 296: 953–55.
- DC C. Agenesis of the vermiform appendix. Am J Surg. 1951; 82: 689–96.
- Shand JE, B.D. Agenesis of the vermiform appendix in a thalidomide child. Br J Surg. 1977; 64: 203–04.
- Ivanschuk G, C.A. S, EP B, C L, M T SR. Amyand's hernia: A review. Med Sci Monit. 2014; 20: 140–46.
- Kronman MP, Z.T. H, K F, R C, S.E. Antibiotic exposure and IBD development among children: A population-based cohort study. Pediatrics. 2012; 130: 794–803.
- Andersson R. Appendectomy and protection against ulcerative colitis. N Engl J Med. 2001; 344: 808–14.
- Sahami S, W.M. K, L. Appendectomy for therapy-refractory ulcerative colitis results in pathological improvement of colonic inflammation: Short-term results of the PASSION study. J Crohns Colitis. 2019; 13: 165171.
- Naganuma M. Appendectomy protects against the development of ulcerative colitis and reduces its recurrence: Results of a multicenter case-controlled study in Japan. Am J Gastroenterol. 2001; 96: 1123–26.
- Rutgeerts P, D.H.G. H, M G, K V, G. Appendectomy protects against ulcerative colitis. Gastroenterology. 1994; 106: 1251–53.
- Nageswaran H, K.U. H, F M, A. Appendiceal duplication: A comprehensive review of published cases and clinical recommendations. World J Surg. 2018; 42: 574–81.
- Bolin TD, W.S. C, R E, JL R, S.M. Appendicectomy as a therapy for ulcerative proctitis. Am J Gastroenterol. 2009; 104: 2476–82.
- Hallas J. Appendicectomy has no beneficial effect on admission rates in patients with ulcerative colitis. Gut. 2004; 53: 351–54.
- DM F. Appendicitis following appendicectomy. J R Coll Surg Edinb. 1984; 29: 61–62.

– Salati SA, R.A. L, NA R, A. Appendicocecal fistula–a rare complication of appendicitis. Online J Health Allied Scs. 2011; 9: 31.
– Schumpelick V, D.B. O, K P, A. Appendix and cecum: Embryology, anatomy, and surgical applications. Surg Clin North Am. 2000; 80: 295–318.
– Matsushita M, T.H. M, Y N, A I, S O, K. Appendix is a priming site in the development of ulcerative colitis. World J Gastroenterol. 2005; 11: 4869–74.
– R F. Appendix situated within thorax. Br J Radiol. 1948; 21: 523–25.
– Akhtar J, E.T. G, E.J. Appendix vermiformis duplex – A lesson for the unwary. Pediatr Surg Int. 1994; 9: 429–30.
– Polese L, B.R. DFG. B1a lymphocytes in the rectal mucosa of ulcerative colitis patients. World J Gastroenterol. 2012; 18: 144–49.
– Gebbers JO, L.J. Bacterial translocation in the normal human appendix parallels the development of the local immune system. Ann NY Acad Sci. 2004; 1029: 337–43.
– Jo G, J.A. Bacterial translocation in the normal human appendix parallels the development of the local immune system. Ann N Y Acad Sci. 2004; 1029: 337–43.
– Lohr J, K.B. C, D A, A.K. Balance of Th1 and Th17 effector and peripheral regulatory T cells. Microbes Infect. 2009; 11: 589–93.
– Bollinger RB, B.A. B, EL L, SS P, W. Biofilms in the large bowel suggest an apparent function of the human vermiform appendix. J Theor Biol. 2007; 249: 826–31.
– Gilbert P, M.A. Biofilms: Their impact on health and their recalcitrance toward biocides. Am J Infect Control. 2001; 29: 252–55.
– Ouattara D, K.Y. B, E S, FG A, HY BN 'Guessan, GG K. et al. Classification of the terminal arterial vascularization of the appendix with a view to its use in reconstruction microsurgery. Surg Radiol Anat. 2007; 29: 635–41.
– Smith HF, F.R. E, ML T, AD B, RR P, W. Comparative anatomy and phylogenetic distribution of the mammalian cecal appendix. J Evol Biol. 2009; 22: 1984–99.
– Greenberg SLL, E.A. M, S. Congenital absence of the vermiform appendix. ANZ J Surg. 2003; 73: 166–67.
– Delayed separation of an appendix-containing umbilical stump. J Pediatr Surg. 1995; 30: 1717–18.
– Wardlaw T, S.P. B, C C, M M, E. Diarrhoea: Why children are still dying and what can be done. Lancet. 2009; 375: 870–72.
– PH. W. Double appendix. Br J Surg. 1962; 50: 346–47.
– KH L. Duplication of the vermiform appendix in an adult patient. Ann R Coll Surg Engl. 2014; 96: 16–17.
– MA I. Ectopic appendix vermiformis located in the right deep gluteal region due to unilateral piriformis agenesis. Surg Radiol Anat. 2019; 41: 141–42.
– Cosnes J. Effects of appendicectomy on the course of ulcerative colitis. Gut. 2002; 51: 803–07.
– Karl JP, Hatch AM, Arcidiacono SM, Pearce SC, Pantoja-Feliciano IG, Doherty LA. Effects of psychological, environmental and physical stressors on the gut microbiota. Front Microbiol. 2018; 9.
– ME J. Fast renewal of the distal colonic mucus layers by the surface goblet cells as measured by in vivo labeling of mucin glycoproteins. Plos One. 2012; 7: 41009.
– DE. B. Functional histology of appendix. Arch Histol Jpn. 1983; 46: 271–92.
– Malas MA, G.A. S, O. Growing of caecum and vermiform appendix during the fetal period. Fetal Diagn Ther. 2001; 16: 173–77.
– Hewitson JP, G.J. M, R.M. Helminth immunoregulation: The role of parasite secreted proteins in modulating host immunity. Mol Biochem Parasitol. 2009; 167: 1–11.
– Jo Y, M.T. YS. Histological and immunological features of appendix in patients with ulcerative colitis. Dig Dis Sci. 2003; 48: 99–108.

- Mesko TW, L.R. B, T. Horseshoe anomaly of the appendix: A previously undescribed entity. Surgery. 1989; 106: 563–66.
- Calota F, V.I. MS. Horseshoe appendix: A extremely rare anomaly. Chirurgia (Bucur). 2010; 105: 271–74.
- Xiang H, H.J. R, WE R, L.J. Horseshoe appendix: Anatomical variant. J Med Imaging Radiat Oncol. 2018; 62: 83.
- Karul M, B.C. K, S T, TY Y, J. Imaging of appendicitis in adults. Rofo. 2014; 186: 551–58.
- Chauhan S, A.S. Intracecal appendix: An extremely rare anatomical variation. A case report and review of literature. Surg Radiol Anat. 2018; 40: 111–14.
- TW S. Langman's Medical Embryology. Baltimore, Williams &: Wilkins, 1985; pp. 224–46.
- Järnerot G. Laparoscopic appendectomy in patients with refractory ulcerative colitis. Gastroenterology. 2001; 120: 1562–63.
- WW B. Lumbar appendicitis and lumbar appendectomy. Surg Gynecol Obstet. 1946; 82: 414–16.
- Stringer MD, S.L. AR. Management of alimentary tract duplication in children. Br J Surg. 1995; 82: 74–78.
- Deng P, W.J. Meta-analysis of the association between appendiceal orifice inflammation and appendectomy and ulcerative colitis. Rev Esp Enferm Dig. 2016; 108: 401–10.
- Costerton JW, L.Z. C, DE K, DR LS, H.M. Microbial biofilms. Annu Rev Microbiol. 1995; 49: 711–45.
- Palestrant D, Holzknecht ZE, Collins BH, Miller SE, Parker W, Bollinger RR. Microbial biofilms in the gut: Visualization by electron microscopy and by acridine orange staining. Ultrastruct Pathol. 2004; 28: 23–27.
- Guinane CM, Tadrous A, Fouhy F, Ryan CA, Dempsey EM, Murphy B. Microbial composition of human appendices from patients following appendectomy. MBio. 2013; 00366–12.
- M. H. Multiple myenteric networks in the human appendix. Auton Neurosci. 2004; 15:110: 49–54.
- Fitzgerald MJT, O'Neil MN. The position of the human caecum in fetal life. J Anat. 1971; 109: 71–74.
- Bulut SP, C.g.N. A, M. Perforated double appendicitis: Horseshoe type. Turkish J Surgery/Ulusal Cerrahi Dergisi. 2016; 32: 134.
- Somekh E, S.F. G, A V, M L, D. Phenotypic pattern of B cells in the appendix: Reduced intensity of CD19 expression. Immunobiology. 2000; 201: 461–69.
- Radford-Smith GL, E.J. PDM. Protective role of appendicectomy on onset and severity of ulcerative colitis and Crohn's disease. Gut. 2002; 51: 808–13.
- Matsushita M, U.K. O, K. Role of the appendix in the pathogenesis of ulcerative colitis. Inflammopharmacology. 2007; 15: 154–57.
- Odze RD, G.J. Surgical Pathology of the GI Tract, Liver, Biliary Tract and Pancreas. Philadelphia: Saunders, 2008.
- Im GY, M.R. LCT. The appendix may protect against *Clostridium difficile* recurrence. Clin Gastroenterol Hepatol. 2011; 9: 1072–77.
- Skandalakis JE, G.S. R, R.R. The appendix, embryology for surgeons. Chapter. 1994; 15: 491535.
- Vitetta L, Vitetta G, Hall S. The brain-intestinal mucosa-appendix- microbiome-brain loop. Diseases. 2018; 6: 23.
- Laurin M, E.M. P, W. The cecal appendix: One more immune component with a function disturbed by post-industrial culture. Anat Rec (Hoboken). 2011; 294: 567–79.
- CR D. The Descent of Man, and Selection in Relation to Sex. 1st edn, London: John Murray, 1871; pp. 27–28.
- Moore KL, P.T. The Developing Human: Clinically Oriented Embryology. 7th edn, Philadelphia: Saunders, 2003.
- Gardenbroek TJ, E.E. P, CI U, DT. D 'Haens, GR. B, W.A. The effect of appendectomy on the course of ulcerative colitis: A systematic review. Colorectal Dis, 2012; 14: 545–53.

- Hattori M, T.T. The Human Intestinal microbiome: A New Frontier of Human Biology. vol. 16, DNA Res, 2009; pp. 1–12.
- Kooij IA, S.S. M, SL B, CJ TV, A.A. The immunology of the vermiform appendix: A review of the literature. Clin Exp Immunol. 2016; 186: 1–9.
- Johansson ME, P.M. P, J V, A H, L H, G.C. The inner of the two Muc2 mucin-dependent mucus layers in colon is devoid of bacteria. Proc Natl Acad Sci USA. 2008; 105: 15064–69.
- WF M. The intramural appendix. Central Afr J Med. 1977; 18: 54–55.
- C DC. The length and position of the vermiform appendix: A study of 4,680 specimens. Ann Surg. 1932; 96: 1044.
- RE F. The primate appendix: A reassessment. Anat Rec. 2000; 261: 228–36.
- S GB. The primate caecum and appendix vermiformis: A comparative study. J Anat. 1980; 131: 549.
- R N. The primate colon. Proc Zool Soc Lond. 1936; 26: 433–53.
- Beneventano TC, S.C. J, H.G. The roentgen aspects of some appendiceal abnormalities. Am J Roentgenol Radium Ther Nucl Med. 1966; 96: 344–60.
- RJ B. The true caecal apex, or the vermiform appendix: Its minute and comparative anatomy. J Anat Physiol. 1900; 35: 83.
- Barlow A, M.M. G, J M, P T, RS L, M. The vermiform appendix: A review. Clin Anat. 2013; 26(7): 833–42.
- RW S, E.D. Q, K U, JF T Jr, R W, J.V. Trichuris suis seems to be safe and possibly effective in the treatment of inflammatory bowel disease. Am J Gastroenterol. 2003; 198: 2034–41.
- Kacprzyk A, D.J. S, T. Variations and morphometric features of the vermiform appendix: A systematic review and meta-analysis of 114,080 subjects with clinical implications. Clin Anat. 2020; 33: 85–98.
- G W. Vergetauschter doppelter wormfortsatz. Zentralblatt Fur Chirurgie. 1930; 57.
- Kelly HA, H.E. Vermiform Appendix and Its Diseases. Philadelphia: WB Saunders, 1905.
- Kim JH, J.Z. S, S M, G H, S RV, J.F. Vermiform appendix during the repackaging process from umbilical herniation to fixation onto the right posterior abdomen: A study of human fetal horizontal sections. Clin Anat. 2020; 33: 667–77.
- DJ A. Vermiform appendix located within the cecal wall. Anomalies and bizarre locations. Dis Colon Rectum. 1983; 26: 386–89.
- K K. Vertebrates: Comparative Anatomy, Function, Evolution. 6th edn, New York: McGraw-Hill, 2012.
- Bickler SW, D.A. Western diseases: Current concepts and implications for pediatric surgery research and practice. Pediatr Surg Int. 2008; 24: 251–55.
- Ansaloni L, C.F. P, A.D. What is the function of the human vermiform appendix?. Evolution-based surgery: A new perspective in the Darwinian year 2009. Eur Surg Res. 2009; 43: 67–71.

Chapter 2
Inflammatory diseases

2.1 Introduction

Acute appendicitis is the most common surgical emergency in the Western world. The lifetime risk of developing this condition is estimated to be around 6–7%, with peak incidence occurring during the second decade of life and a slight predominance in males. Some studies have suggested a declining trend in cases in recent years, though no definitive explanation has been identified. The decline is likely due to improved hygiene, dietary changes, and medical advancements. Better sanitation and lower childhood infection rates reduce lymphoid hyperplasia, a key trigger of appendicitis. Increased fiber intake prevents fecalith formation, while widespread antibiotic use may resolve early infections before they progress. Advances in imaging allow early diagnosis and conservative treatment, reducing severe cases. Additionally, shifts in the gut microbiome and a growing preference for nonsurgical management contribute to this trend. The interplay of these factors has led to a steady decrease in appendicitis, especially in high-income countries.

Seasonal variations have been observed in several studies, indicating a higher incidence of acute appendicitis during the summer months. Heat-related immune modulation may also play a role, as seasonal variations affect immune responses and gut microbiota composition. Additionally, lifestyle changes during summer, including increased travel and outdoor activities, might contribute to delayed medical attention, leading to more diagnosed cases. Geographical differences in the incidence of acute appendicitis are influenced by a combination of environmental, dietary, socioeconomic, and healthcare-related factors. In high-income countries, lower infection rates due to improved hygiene, widespread antibiotic use, and higher fiber intake have contributed to a declining incidence. In contrast, low- and middle-income countries (LMICs) still experience higher rates, likely due to increased exposure to enteric infections, lower sanitation standards, and diets that may promote fecalith formation. Climate also plays a role – warmer regions often see higher seasonal spikes, possibly due to dehydration and infection prevalence. Additionally, healthcare accessibility affects reported incidence; regions with advanced diagnostic tools may detect more mild cases, while areas with limited access might underreport or diagnose only severe cases. These factors collectively shape the geographical variations observed in appendicitis rates worldwide.

Despite its high prevalence in developed countries, diagnosing appendicitis remains challenging due to the lack of highly specific and reliable distinguishing features. Clinical scoring systems have been developed to aid in diagnosis and management, yet clinical judgment continues to play a crucial role in decision-making. Despite advancements in imaging and laboratory testing, clinical judgment remains

https://doi.org/10.1515/9783112219782-002

critical in diagnosing acute appendicitis due to the variability in presentation and the limitations of diagnostic tools. Symptoms can be atypical, especially in children, the elderly, and pregnant women, requiring a careful history and physical examination to guide decision-making. While ultrasound and CT scans improve accuracy, they are not always definitive, and overreliance on imaging can delay treatment. Experienced clinicians assess symptom progression, response to palpation (e.g., McBurney's point tenderness and rebound pain), and laboratory markers to make timely decisions, especially in settings with limited access to imaging. Moreover, appendicitis mimics several other conditions (e.g., gastroenteritis, ovarian pathology, and diverticulitis), making clinical expertise essential to avoid misdiagnosis and unnecessary surgery. Ultimately, a balanced approach combining clinical acumen with diagnostic tools ensures optimal patient outcomes.

The first documented appendectomy was performed in 1735 by Claudius Amyand on a patient with a strangulated inguinal hernia, whose hernia sac contained the appendix. In 1759, the French physician Mestier is believed to have performed the first appendectomy specifically for acute appendicitis. However, the first comprehensive description of the disease and the recommendation for surgical removal of the appendix are credited to Reginald Heber Fitz of Harvard University. In a remarkable case, 27-year-old Leonid Rogozov performed an appendectomy on himself on April 30, 1961, while stranded with a Soviet expedition team in Antarctica. As the only doctor on the expedition, he had no choice but to operate on himself in order to remove his inflamed appendix. With the assistance of a meteorologist and a driver – who handed him instruments and held a mirror – Rogozov performed the surgery under local anesthesia, using only a mirror and touch to guide himself. The operation lasted about 2 h, and despite the challenging conditions, he successfully removed his appendix. He recovered quickly and resumed his duties after 2 weeks.

Key advancements in the management of appendicitis include McBurney's introduction of the classic muscle-splitting incision technique for appendectomy in 1894 and Kurt Semm's first laparoscopic appendectomy in 1982. Today, laparoscopic appendectomy is the standard of care when surgical intervention is required. In children, acute appendicitis is the most common indication for emergency abdominal surgery. Morbidity remains significant in this population, with an overall appendix perforation rate of 12.5–30%. The high rate of appendix perforation in children with acute appendicitis is primarily due to a combination of delayed diagnosis, anatomical differences, and rapid disease progression. Young children often struggle to accurately describe their symptoms, leading to misinterpretation and delays in seeking medical attention. Additionally, their immune response is immature, and their omentum, which in adults helps contain infection, is underdeveloped, allowing inflammation to spread more quickly. The appendix itself has a thinner wall in children, making it more prone to rupture once inflamed. Moreover, appendicitis in this age group frequently presents with nonspecific or atypical symptoms, such as diffuse abdominal pain, vomiting, or irritability rather than the classic right lower quadrant pain seen in older patients. This contributes to frequent misdiagnosis, further delaying treatment. Since the disease progresses rapidly, often leading to perforation within 24–48 h of symptom onset, early imaging and a high index of suspicion are crucial to prevent complications.

Ongoing debates and controversies continue to shape the diagnosis, treatment, and management of appendicitis. Research is focused on optimizing diagnostic testing, determining the role of antibiotic therapy versus appendectomy, evaluating the best surgical approach (minimally invasive vs. open surgery), defining an acceptable negative appendectomy rate, managing intraoperative findings of appendiceal masses, and addressing the unique considerations of special populations such as pregnant women, the elderly, and immunosuppressed patients.

2.2 Pathophysiology and differential diagnosis

The primary mechanism underlying the pathogenesis of appendicitis is luminal obstruction, a common event due to the slender diameter of the appendix. This narrow aperture plays a physiological role in providing shelter for beneficial bacteria and facilitating biofilm formation. However, when obstruction occurs, mucus produced by the epithelial lining and gas formed by bacterial activity accumulate within the limited space, leading to increased intraluminal pressure. Concurrently, bacterial overgrowth is facilitated by the obstruction, which is particularly relevant in cases of perforated appendicitis, as it results in the release of a larger bacterial inoculum into the peritoneal cavity. The progressive rise in pressure against the appendix wall eventually reaches venous pressure, preventing venous blood return and leading to ischemia of the appendiceal tissue. If left unresolved, full-thickness ischemia ensues, culminating in perforation and subsequent peritonitis. The time from obstruction onset to perforation varies widely, ranging from a few hours to several days. The clinical outcomes following perforation are equally variable, with peri-appendiceal or pelvic abscesses forming in some cases, while in others, free perforation leads to diffuse peritonitis. In certain instances, the omentum and adjacent viscera wall off the inflamed appendix, forming an inflammatory mass that can obscure classic symptoms. Some minor episodes of mucosal inflammation may resolve spontaneously, potentially explaining reports of transient, self-limiting abdominal pain in patients with acute appendicitis.

As previously discussed, the bacterial flora of the appendix closely resembles that of the colon, making appendicitis-associated infections polymicrobial. Broad-spectrum antibiotics should be administered to cover both gram-positive and gram-negative bacteria. Several factors contribute to luminal obstruction, including fecal stasis, fecaliths, lymphoid hyperplasia, neoplasms, fruit and vegetable material, ingested barium, and parasitic infections such as *Ascaris lumbricoides.* A fecalith is found in approximately 20% of children with acute appendicitis. Carras et al. suggested prophylactic appendectomy in cases where an appendicolith is visible on plain radiographs. Forbes and Lloyd-Davies classified appendicoliths based on calcium content into noncalcified fecal pellets, partially calcified fecaliths, and fully calcified stony calculi, recommending appendectomy when an appendicolith is incidentally detected on radiological examination due to its association with complicated appendicitis. However, appendectomy should not be performed solely based on the incidental finding of a fecalith on a plain radiograph. The presence of a fecalith alone is not diagnostic of acute appendicitis, and many individuals with fecaliths remain asymptomatic throughout their lives without ever developing inflammation. While it is true that fecaliths are a known risk factor for appendicitis, their mere presence does not justify surgical intervention in the absence of clinical symptoms.

While no specific genetic causes of acute appendicitis have been identified, studies in twins and individuals with a positive family history suggest an increased risk. The development of appendicitis is generally considered multifactorial, involving a combination of luminal obstruction, bacterial proliferation, and host immune response. However, there is increasing evidence suggesting a genetic predisposition to appendicitis, though no single gene has been definitively identified as the cause.

Several studies have demonstrated a familial tendency for appendicitis, with first-degree relatives of affected individuals having a higher risk of developing the condition. Twin studies have further supported a genetic component, as monozygotic twins show a higher concordance rate for appendicitis compared to dizygotic twins. Additionally, certain genetic polymorphisms related to immune function, inflammation, and susceptibility to infections have been proposed as potential contributors. Variants in genes involved in innate immunity, such as those encoding cytokines and toll-like receptors, may influence an individual's inflammatory response and predisposition to appendiceal inflammation.

Ethnic and geographical variations in the incidence of appendicitis also suggest a potential genetic influence, although dietary and environmental factors play a significant role. While genetic predisposition may contribute to an individual's susceptibility, appendicitis remains largely a condition triggered by obstructive and inflammatory processes rather than a purely hereditary disease.

Interestingly, some researchers argue that perforation is not solely due to elevated intraluminal pressure. Traditionally, the progression of appendicitis to perforation has been attributed to obstruction of the appendiceal lumen, leading to increased pressure, ischemia, and eventual necrosis of the appendiceal wall. However, recent studies measuring luminal pressure in patients with appendicitis have challenged this notion, finding that elevated pressure is present in only a quarter of cases. This suggests that factors beyond mechanical obstruction play a significant role in determining whether an inflamed appendix will perforate.

Emerging evidence supports the idea that perforated and nonperforated appendicitis may represent distinct clinical entities rather than different stages of the same disease process. For example, some studies have observed that patients who present with perforation often have a longer duration of symptoms but not necessarily more severe initial pain, implying that their appendicitis may follow a different pathological course. Furthermore, there are indications that host immune response plays a critical role in determining whether an inflamed appendix will perforate. Patients with altered inflammatory responses, such as those with genetic polymorphisms affecting cytokine production, may be predisposed to more aggressive forms of appendicitis.

Another growing area of research focuses on the role of the colonic microbiome in the progression of appendicitis. Differences in microbial composition have been noted between patients with perforated and nonperforated appendicitis, suggesting that specific bacterial populations may contribute to either a controlled or a more destructive inflammatory response. Some studies have found an overrepresentation of pathogenic bacteria in perforated cases, while others have highlighted a depletion of beneficial commensal microbes that might otherwise regulate inflammation. These findings raise the possibility that appendicitis, particularly its progression to perforation, may be influenced by dysbiosis rather than purely mechanical factors.

These findings collectively challenge the long-held notion that perforation is merely a consequence of unchecked luminal pressure, suggesting instead that a complex interplay of immune response, microbial factors, and genetic predisposition may contribute to disease progression. This paradigm shift underscores the necessity of a more nuanced and multifactorial approach to understanding the pathophysiology of appendiceal perforation. Future research directions may include the identification of specific biomarkers that can reliably predict perforation risk, allowing for early intervention and tailored management strategies. Additionally, growing evidence points to the gut microbiome as a key player in appendiceal inflammation and perforation, prompting interest in microbiome-targeted therapies such as probiotics, prebiotics, or even fecal microbiota transplantation as potential preventative or therapeutic interventions. Furthermore, refining existing treatment algorithms by incorporating personalized risk stratification models could help optimize surgical and nonsurgical approaches, ultimately reducing complications and improving patient outcomes in high-risk populations.

A debated theory proposes classifying acute appendicitis into different patterns of inflammation with distinct pathophysiologies. One form, termed "simple appendicitis," is characterized by inflammation without tissue necrosis and may not progress to perforation. This milder variant may resolve spontaneously or be managed conservatively with antibiotics. In contrast, "complicated appendicitis" progresses rapidly to gangrene and perforation. Evidence supporting this theory includes microbiological differences between uncomplicated and complicated cases and distinct epidemiological trends. Emerging research indicates that individual variations in immune response play a significant role in determining the severity and clinical course of appendicitis. Specifically, studies suggest that a predominance of Th1-mediated immune responses is associated with complicated cases, including gangrenous or perforated appendicitis, likely due to an exaggerated proinflammatory cytokine release that drives extensive tissue damage. In contrast, Th2-mediated immune responses appear to be linked to milder, uncomplicated forms of the disease, potentially due to a more balanced inflammatory reaction that limits excessive tissue destruction. These findings highlight the importance of immunological profiling in appendicitis and open new avenues for personalized therapeutic strategies. Future research may explore the potential of modulating immune pathways to prevent progression to severe forms as well as identifying biomarkers that could aid in early risk stratification and targeted intervention.

Despite a clinical presentation consistent with acute appendicitis, a notable proportion of appendectomy specimens fail to demonstrate histological evidence of inflammation, raising questions about alternative pathogenic mechanisms. Interestingly, many of these patients experience symptom resolution following surgical removal of the appendix, suggesting that factors beyond overt inflammation may contribute to their clinical presentation. As early as 1910, Maresh and Masson proposed that neuroendocrine alterations could lead to appendiceal pain in the absence of detectable inflammation.

Subsequent research has supported this hypothesis by identifying neuroproliferation and increased expression of neuropeptides such as substance P (SP) and vasoactive intestinal peptide (VIP) in patients with negative histology. These neuropeptides, known for their roles in nociception and inflammatory modulation, may be key contributors to the right lower quadrant pain characteristic of appendicitis. Neurogenic inflammation, driven by SP and VIP, is believed to induce localized pain, vasodilation, and increased vascular permeability, mimicking the effects of classical inflammation.

Additionally, studies have revealed neuronal hypertrophy in histologically normal appendices, a finding reminiscent of alterations observed in inflammatory bowel diseases (IBDs), further supporting the role of neural mechanisms in appendiceal pain. Beyond neurogenic factors, increased expression of inflammatory mediators such as cyclooxygenases, prostaglandins, nitric oxide synthase, and major histocompatibility complex class II molecules has been detected in both inflamed and histologically normal appendices. This suggests the presence of subtle, molecular-level inflammatory processes that may not be apparent through standard histopathological examination.

These insights challenge the traditional binary classification of appendicitis as either inflammatory or noninflammatory and highlight the need for a broader perspective incorporating neuroimmune interactions. Future studies should aim to refine diagnostic criteria, explore targeted therapies modulating neurogenic inflammation, and assess whether certain subsets of patients with appendiceal pain might benefit from nonsurgical management strategies.

A subset of appendicitis cases has been linked to amebiasis, a parasitic infection caused by *Entamoeba histolytica*, which predominantly affects the colon but can also involve the appendix. In these cases, appendiceal inflammation may result from luminal obstruction due to mucosal edema triggered by the presence of trophozoites, the active and invasive form of the parasite. The transmission of *E. histolytica* occurs primarily through the ingestion of cysts in contaminated food or water, with humans acting as the main reservoir for the parasite.

While amebic appendicitis can coexist with amebic dysentery – classically presenting as diarrhea with mucus and blood – many patients exhibit no overt gastrointestinal symptoms. In fact, the clinical presentation of amebic appendicitis often mimics that of typical bacterial appendicitis, making diagnosis challenging. A study by Guzman and Valdivia reported that only 2.3% of patients with amebic appendicitis showed signs of dysentery, suggesting that appendiceal involvement can occur even in the absence of widespread colonic disease. This underscores the need for a high index of suspicion in endemic regions or in patients with risk factors such as travel history or immunosuppression.

Histopathological examination of resected appendices often reveals trophozoites within the inflamed mucosa, sometimes extending into the submucosa and muscular layers, leading to necrotizing inflammation. In severe cases, extensive tissue destruction may predispose to perforation. Given the potential for misdiagnosis, clinicians should consider stool antigen testing, serology, or PCR-based methods to identify *E. histolytica* in suspected cases.

Management of amebic appendicitis typically involves appendectomy combined with antiparasitic therapy, such as metronidazole, to eradicate systemic infection and prevent recurrence. Unlike bacterial appendicitis, where surgery alone is often curative, failure to address the underlying parasitic infection can lead to persistent colonic disease or extraintestinal complications such as liver abscesses. Future research should aim to improve diagnostic methods and assess the long-term outcomes of patients with amebic appendicitis, particularly in endemic regions.

The pain experienced in acute appendicitis arises from a combination of visceral and somatic sensory pathways, reflecting the progression of the inflammatory process. In the early stages, visceral pain originates from distension, ischemia, or irritation of the appendix itself. This discomfort is typically vague, dull, and poorly localized to the periumbilical or epigastric region due to the transmission of autonomic afferent signals via unmyelinated C fibers to the dorsal root ganglia of the lower thoracic spinal cord (T8–T10). This early phase of pain is characteristic of many intra-abdominal visceral processes, making diagnosis challenging.

As appendiceal inflammation worsens and extends to involve the adjacent parietal peritoneum, the pain undergoes a distinct transition. The somatic pain fibers of the parietal peritoneum, which are carried by the lower intercostal and lumbar nerves, provide precise localization and sharper pain perception. This shift results in the classic migration of pain from the periumbilical region to the right iliac fossa, a hallmark feature of acute appendicitis. Unlike visceral pain, which is diffuse and difficult to pinpoint, somatic pain is well-localized and exacerbated by movement, deep palpation, or peritoneal irritation, as seen in signs such as rebound tenderness and guarding.

The dual nature of appendiceal pain underscores the importance of careful clinical assessment, as it reflects the complex interplay between visceral and somatic pain pathways. Initially, the pain is often vague and poorly localized, originating from the midline periumbilical region due to visceral innervation shared with the midgut. As inflammation progresses and involves the parietal peritoneum, the pain typically shifts to the right lower quadrant, becoming sharper and more localized – this transition being a hallmark of appendicitis. However, variability in pain localization can occur, particularly in cases of retrocecal or pelvic appendices. A retrocecal appendix, which is positioned behind the cecum, may lead to a less pronounced anterior abdominal pain response due to the protective effect of the overlying bowel, sometimes manifesting instead as flank or back pain. Conversely, a pelvic appendix, extending downward into the pelvis, may irritate adjacent structures such as the bladder or rectum, leading to urinary symptoms, tenesmus, or deep pelvic discomfort rather than the classic McBurney's point tenderness. These anatomical variations can obscure the diagnosis and necessitate a higher degree of clinical suspicion.

In elderly or immunocompromised patients, the classic presentation of appendicitis can be significantly altered, making diagnosis more challenging. The typical evolution of appendiceal pain, which usually transitions from a vague, visceral discomfort to a more localized somatic pain in the right lower quadrant, may be blunted or entirely absent. This phenomenon can be attributed to several physiological factors, including age-related changes in the immune system, underlying neuropathy, and diminished pain perception. In elderly patients, a general decline in inflammatory response can result in a more indolent disease course, while in immunocompromised individuals – such as those undergoing chemotherapy, receiving immunosuppressive therapy for organ transplantation, or living with conditions like diabetes or HIV – the inflammatory cascade may be inadequate to trigger the usual pain patterns and systemic signs of infection.

As a consequence, these patients may present with atypical symptoms such as mild abdominal discomfort, anorexia, generalized weakness, or low-grade fever rather than the hallmark signs of acute appendicitis. Some may experience only nonspecific gastrointestinal symptoms, including nausea, bloating, or altered bowel habits, which can be mistakenly attributed to other chronic conditions, delaying the recognition of an evolving intra-abdominal emergency. Additionally, cognitive impairment in elderly patients, such as in those with dementia, may further obscure the clinical picture by limiting their ability to accurately describe symptoms.

The delayed or atypical presentation in these vulnerable populations significantly increases the risk of complications. Without the usual early warning signs prompting timely medical intervention, the appendix may continue to inflame and progress to perforation before the diagnosis is established. This, in turn, raises the likelihood of localized or diffuse peritonitis, abscess formation, and, ultimately, sepsis, all of which are associated with higher morbidity and mortality rates in these high-risk groups. Therefore, a high index of suspicion and a lower threshold for advanced imaging, such as CT scanning, are crucial in evaluating elderly and immunocompromised patients with unexplained abdominal symptoms to ensure prompt diagnosis and timely surgical or medical management.

Understanding these pain pathways not only aids in early recognition of appendicitis but also provides crucial insight into atypical presentations. Physicians must remain vigilant in cases where the clinical picture deviates from textbook descriptions, employing advanced imaging modalities such as ultrasound, CT, or MRI when necessary. A high index of suspicion, particularly in high-risk populations or those with anatomical variations, ensures timely intervention and reduces morbidity associated with delayed diagnosis.

Given its variable presentation, appendicitis should be considered in all patients with acute abdominal pain. Differential diagnoses vary by age, sex, and clinical history. In children, mesenteric adenitis, gastroenteritis, intussusception, Meckel's diverticulitis, IBD, and testicular torsion must be considered. Nephrolithiasis and urinary tract infections (UTIs) may also mimic appendicitis. In women of reproductive age, alternative diagnoses include ruptured ovarian cysts, ovulation pain (mittelschmerz), endometriosis, ovarian torsion, ectopic pregnancy, and pelvic inflammatory disease (PID). In elderly patients, diverticulitis and malignancies are common causes of lower abdominal pain, while in immunocompromised individuals, neutropenic enterocolitis is a crucial consideration.

Other conditions mimicking appendicitis include:

– **Gastroenteritis**: Gastroenteritis is a common condition that typically presents with diarrhea as the predominant symptom before the onset of abdominal pain, distinguishing it from appendicitis, in which pain usually precedes gastrointestinal symptoms. The presence of fever, nausea, vomiting, and diffuse crampy abdominal discomfort further supports a diagnosis of infectious gastroenteritis rather than an acute surgical abdomen. However, in some cases, particularly with bacterial pathogens, the presentation can closely mimic appendicitis, leading to diagnostic uncertainty.

One such pathogen is *Yersinia enterocolitica*, a gram-negative bacterium that causes mesenteric adenitis, an inflammatory condition affecting the lymph nodes in the ileocecal region. Infection with *Yersinia* can closely resemble acute appendicitis, as it often produces right lower quadrant pain, fever, and leukocytosis. Unlike true appendicitis, however, patients with *Yersinia* infection typically exhibit a preceding or concurrent diarrheal illness, which can aid in differentiation. The infection is more common in children and young adults and may be associated with exposure to contaminated food, particularly undercooked pork, unpasteurized dairy products, or untreated water.

Given the clinical overlap between *Yersinia* infection and appendicitis, accurate diagnosis requires laboratory testing. Stool cultures remain the primary diagnostic tool, as *Yersinia* can be isolated from fecal samples, although the bacteria require specific culture conditions for optimal detection. In cases where stool cultures are negative or inconclusive, serologic testing for anti-*Yersinia* antibodies can provide additional diagnostic confirmation, especially in patients with prolonged or recurrent symptoms. In some instances, imaging studies, such as ultrasound or CT scans, may reveal enlarged mesenteric lymph nodes, further suggesting an infectious rather than a surgical etiology.

Although *Yersinia* infections are generally self-limiting, severe or complicated cases – such as those in immunocompromised individuals – may warrant antibiotic treatment with agents like fluoroquinolones or trimethoprim-sulfamethoxazole. Awareness of this potential appendicitis mimic is crucial to avoid unnecessary appendectomies and to ensure appropriate management, particularly in endemic areas or at-risk populations.

– **Urinary tract infection**: (UTI should be considered in patients presenting with dysuria, urinary frequency, urgency, or suprapubic discomfort, particularly in the absence of significant gastrointestinal symptoms. In female patients, in whom UTIs are more common due to a shorter urethra, distinguishing between a lower UTI and other causes of abdominal or pelvic pain is crucial. While UTIs often present with localized urinary symptoms, upper urinary tract involvement (pyelonephritis) can cause flank pain, fever, and systemic signs, which may further complicate the differential diagnosis when considering acute appendicitis.

Urinalysis and urine culture are essential diagnostic tools in evaluating a suspected UTI. The presence of pyuria (white blood cells (WBCs) in the urine), bacteriuria, and, in some cases, hematuria supports the diagnosis, while urine culture helps identify the causative organism and guide antibiotic therapy. However, a UTI does not necessarily exclude the presence of appendicitis, as inflammation of the appendix – especially when located near the bladder or ureter – can cause secondary urinary symptoms, such as dysuria or mild urinary frequency, due to local irritation. Additionally, appendiceal inflammation can sometimes lead to sterile pyuria, where WBCs are present in the urine without an actual bacterial infection, further confounding the clinical picture.

In cases where diagnostic uncertainty remains, imaging studies such as abdominal ultrasound or computed tomography (CT) scan are valuable in differentiating between appendicitis and a primary UTI, particularly in patients with overlapping symptoms. Recognizing that UTIs and appendicitis can coexist or mimic each other is crucial to prevent misdiagnosis and ensure timely and appropriate treatment:

– **Gynecologic conditions**: Gynecologic conditions must always be considered in the differential diagnosis of right lower quadrant pain, particularly in female patients of reproductive age. Conditions such as ruptured ovarian cysts, PID due to tubal infections, and ectopic pregnancies can closely mimic appendicitis, necessitating thorough gynecologic evaluation to ensure accurate diagnosis and appropriate management.

A ruptured ovarian cyst can present with sudden-onset, sharp pelvic pain, which may be localized to the right lower quadrant if the affected ovary is on that side. The pain may be accompanied by mild vaginal bleeding due to hormonal changes or peritoneal irritation from cyst fluid or blood. Unlike appendicitis, which typically progresses over hours, ovarian cyst rupture is often abrupt and may follow physical activity or sexual intercourse. While small cysts resolve spontaneously, larger hemorrhagic cysts can cause significant intra-abdominal bleeding, requiring surgical intervention.

PID, commonly caused by sexually transmitted infections such as *Chlamydia trachomatis* or *Neisseria gonorrhoeae*, often presents with lower abdominal pain, fever, and cervical motion tenderness on pelvic examination. Inflammation of the fallopian tubes (salpingitis) can lead to peritoneal irritation, mimicking the localized pain of appendicitis. Additional symptoms such as abnormal vaginal discharge, dyspareunia, and menstrual irregularities help distinguish PID from surgical causes. Left untreated, PID may result in complications such as tubo-ovarian abscesses and infertility, underscoring the importance of early recognition and antibiotic therapy.

Ectopic pregnancy is a life-threatening condition that must be ruled out in any woman of childbearing age presenting with lower abdominal pain, particularly if accompanied by amenorrhea or abnormal vaginal bleeding. An ectopic pregnancy occurs when a fertilized egg implants outside the uterine cavity, most commonly in the fallopian tube. As the pregnancy progresses, tubal distension or rupture can cause severe pain and intra-abdominal bleeding, leading to hemodynamic instability in severe cases. A positive pregnancy test, coupled with transvaginal ultrasound findings showing an empty uterus despite elevated β-hCG levels, is diagnostic. Prompt identification is crucial, as untreated ectopic pregnancy can rapidly progress to hemorrhagic shock, necessitating urgent medical or surgical intervention.

Given the overlapping symptoms of these gynecologic conditions with appendicitis, a comprehensive clinical assessment, including pelvic examination, β-hCG testing, and pelvic ultrasound, is essential. Failure to consider these alternative diagnoses may lead to unnecessary appendectomy or, conversely, delayed treatment of a potentially life-threatening gynecologic emergency:

– **Intestinal obstruction**: Intestinal obstruction is an important consideration in the differential diagnosis of abdominal pain, particularly in patients presenting with nausea, vomiting, abdominal distension, and constipation or obstipation. Mechanical obstruction can result from various causes, including adhesions, hernias, malignancies, volvulus, or inflammatory conditions such as Crohn's disease. Functional obstruction, or ileus, occurs due to impaired bowel motility and can be triggered by intra-abdominal infections, electrolyte imbalances, or recent surgery.

Radiologic imaging is essential in distinguishing true mechanical obstruction from other causes of abdominal pain. Abdominal X-rays may reveal dilated bowel loops with air-fluid levels, suggestive of an obstructive process. However, CT with contrast provides a more definitive assessment, identifying the site, severity, and potential cause of the obstruction while also ruling out other conditions such as appendicitis, neoplasms, or intra-abdominal abscesses.

Perforated appendicitis can complicate the clinical picture by inducing a paralytic ileus, mimicking mechanical obstruction. When the appendix perforates, localized peritonitis and inflammation can lead to bowel dysmotility, causing diffuse abdominal distension, decreased bowel sounds, and failure to pass flatus or stool. In such cases, CT imaging may show free air, peritoneal fluid, or an abscess, distinguishing perforated appendicitis from a primary obstruction.

Given the overlapping symptoms between intestinal obstruction and appendicitis-related ileus, clinicians must maintain a high index of suspicion and utilize imaging promptly to ensure accurate diagnosis and appropriate management. While true mechanical obstruction may require bowel decompression or surgical intervention, appendiceal perforation with ileus often necessitates antibiotics, fluid resuscitation, and, in most cases, surgical drainage or appendectomy:

– **Constipation**: Constipation is a common gastrointestinal condition that can present with abdominal pain, bloating, and discomfort, sometimes mimicking more serious intra-abdominal pathologies including appendicitis. In severe cases, retained stool can lead to significant colonic distension increased intraluminal pressure, and crampy abdominal pain. The pain is often diffuse or localized to the lower abdomen and is typically relieved by defecation, distinguishing it from acute surgical conditions where pain tends to persist or worsen over time.

Patients with constipation may also experience nausea, decreased appetite, and a sensation of incomplete evacuation. The causes of constipation range from dietary factors (low fiber intake, inadequate hydration) to functional disorders (slow colonic transit, irritable bowel syndrome), medication side effects (opioids, anticholinergics), or underlying medical conditions such as hypothyroidism and neurological disorders.

A careful history, including bowel habits, diet, and medication use, is crucial in differentiating constipation-related pain from acute appendicitis. Physical examination may reveal a palpable fecal mass in the left lower quadrant or generalized tenderness without peritoneal signs. When uncertainty remains, abdominal X-rays can help identify significant fecal loading, while a CT scan may be necessary to exclude other causes of right lower quadrant pain.

Although constipation itself is benign, prolonged or severe cases can lead to complications such as fecal impaction or stercoral colitis, which may require medical intervention. Importantly, constipation does not exclude the possibility of appendicitis, as early appendiceal inflammation may coexist with reduced bowel motility. Therefore, in patients with persistent or worsening pain despite bowel movements, further evaluation is warranted to rule out an underlying surgical cause:

– **Inflammatory bowel disease**: IBD, particularly *Crohn's disease* affecting the termi-nal ileum, can closely mimic acute appendicitis due to its overlapping symptoms in-cluding right lower quadrant pain, fever, nausea, and leukocytosis. The inflammation of the ileum in Crohn's disease, known as ileitis, can present with crampy abdominal pain and tenderness that may be difficult to distinguish from appendiceal inflamma-tion. Additionally, patients with Crohn's disease often experience chronic diarrhea, weight loss, and periods of symptom exacerbation and remission, which can provide important clues to the diagnosis.

Unlike appendicitis, which typically has an acute onset and a progressive course leading to perforation if untreated, *Crohn's disease* tends to have a more protracted presentation, often with prior episodes of similar abdominal pain. In some cases, Crohn's-related inflammation may lead to complications such as strictures, abscess formation, or fistulas, further complicating the clinical picture.

Colonoscopy with ileoscopy and biopsy is essential for the definitive diagnosis of *Crohn's disease*, as it allows direct visualization of the inflamed bowel mucosa, identi-fication of characteristic findings such as skip lesions and cobblestoning, and histo-logic confirmation of chronic inflammation. However, colonoscopy is generally avoided in the acute setting if appendicitis or perforation is strongly suspected due to the risk of exacerbating inflammation or causing perforation. In such cases, imaging studies such as CT or MRI enterography can provide valuable diagnostic information by revealing bowel wall thickening, mesenteric fat stranding, and the presence of strictures or fistulas.

Given the potential for diagnostic confusion, particularly in young patients presenting with right lower quadrant pain, clinicians must consider *Crohn's disease* in the differ-ential diagnosis of suspected appendicitis. Misdiagnosis can lead to unnecessary ap-pendectomy, and while surgery is sometimes needed for Crohn's-related complica-tions, medical management with corticosteroids, immunosuppressants, or biologic therapy is the mainstay of treatment. Therefore, a high index of suspicion and appro-priate use of imaging and endoscopic evaluation are crucial in distinguishing these two conditions and guiding appropriate management.

Recognizing these alternative diagnoses is critical to avoid unnecessary surgery and ensure appropriate management of acute abdominal pain. While appendicitis re-mains one of the most common surgical emergencies, a variety of conditions – includ-ing gastrointestinal, gynecologic, urologic, and systemic diseases – can present with similar symptoms. Misdiagnosis can lead to inappropriate surgical intervention, de-lays in treating the underlying cause, or missed opportunities for conservative man-agement when appropriate.

A thorough history, including symptom onset, progression, associated gastrointes-tinal or urinary symptoms, and any prior similar episodes, is essential in narrowing the differential diagnosis. Physical examination findings, while helpful, may not al-ways be definitive, particularly in elderly, immunocompromised, or pregnant patients, who may present with atypical symptoms. Therefore, laboratory tests such as complete blood count, inflammatory markers, urinalysis, and pregnancy testing in women of reproductive age are crucial adjuncts in the initial evaluation.

Imaging plays a pivotal role in distinguishing appendicitis from its mimics. While ultrasound is a useful first-line tool, especially in pediatric and pregnant patients, CT remains the gold standard for diagnosing appendicitis and identifying alternative causes of right lower quadrant pain, such as IBD, mesenteric adenitis, or gynecologic pathology. In select cases, MRI or colonoscopy may be necessary for further evaluation.

Ultimately, an accurate diagnosis ensures that patients receive timely and appropriate treatment, whether surgical, medical, or conservative. A high index of suspicion for alternative diagnoses, combined with a systematic diagnostic approach, helps reduce the risk of unnecessary appendectomy while preventing delays in managing conditions that require urgent intervention, such as ectopic pregnancy, bowel obstruction, or perforated viscus.

2.3 Clinical presentation

At an early stage, patients with acute appendicitis typically experience vague abdominal pain, often referred to the periumbilical region. This occurs because only visceral afferent fibers are initially stimulated. Accompanying symptoms, such as vomiting and anorexia, may not always be present. As the condition progresses and the tip of the appendix becomes inflamed, the peritoneum covering it gets involved, leading to localized pain in the right lower quadrant. This phenomenon of pain migration is a reliable symptom of appendicitis and is considered pathognomonic.

However, the classic presentation does not always apply, as acute appendicitis can manifest in less typical ways. In fact, the characteristic sequence of periumbilical pain migrating to the right iliac fossa, accompanied by nausea, vomiting, and anorexia, occurs in fewer than half of patients. For example, individuals with retrocecal appendices often present with milder symptoms. If the appendix tip is located in the pelvis, the condition may mimic UTI. In such cases, high clinical suspicion and further diagnostic testing are required to avoid missing the diagnosis.

The duration of clinical symptoms varies, typically ranging from 24 to 48 h, though it can extend beyond 5 days in cases of an appendiceal mass. Patients usually remain still in bed, as movement exacerbates pain due to peritoneal involvement. Mild fever is commonly observed, but its absence does not exclude the diagnosis. Fever severity can vary depending on disease progression and the intensity of the inflammatory response. Dehydration and tachycardia may develop, with the latter resulting from fever, hypotension, and a sympathetic response to pain.

Abdominal examination usually reveals tenderness and guarding in the right iliac fossa. Rebound tenderness suggests localized peritonitis. Diffuse abdominal rigidity with absent peristalsis indicates involuntary muscular spasm, raising suspicion of perforation. Several clinical signs can support the diagnosis of acute appendicitis by detecting localized peritonitis through specific maneuvers.

2.3.1 McBurney sign

It is named after Charles McBurney, an American surgeon who, in the late nineteenth century, described the precise anatomical location of the appendix in relation to abdominal pain. This sign is one of the most widely recognized physical examination techniques for evaluating suspected appendicitis and is a key component of the diagnostic process.

McBurney's point, the focal area for this sign, is located in the right lower quadrant of the abdomen. It is identified as a spot approximately one-third of the distance from the anterior superior iliac spine (ASIS), a bony prominence on the pelvis, to the umbilicus (belly button). This point corresponds to the typical location of the base of the appendix, making it a critical landmark during physical examination.

To assess McBurney's sign, a healthcare provider applies firm pressure to McBurney's point. If the patient experiences significant tenderness or pain at this location, the sign is considered positive. This tenderness is often a result of inflammation or irritation of the appendix, which is located deep beneath this point. In some cases, the pain may intensify when the pressure is suddenly released, a phenomenon known as rebound tenderness, which further supports the diagnosis of appendicitis. This happens because the peritoneum, which is already inflamed or irritated, is stretched or moved during the release of pressure. When the abdominal wall springs back into place, the movement aggravates the sensitive peritoneum, leading to a sudden and intense pain response. This phenomenon is distinct from the pain felt during direct palpation and is a hallmark of peritoneal irritation.

The significance of McBurney's sign lies in its ability to localize the source of abdominal pain to the appendix. However, it is important to note that the position of the appendix can vary slightly among individuals, and in some cases, the appendix may be located in atypical positions, such as retrocecal (behind the cecum) or pelvic. These variations can sometimes make the interpretation of McBurney's sign less straightforward.

McBurney's sign is rarely used in isolation for diagnosis. It is typically combined with other clinical findings, such as Rovsing's sign, obturator sign, psoas sign, and laboratory or imaging studies like blood tests, ultrasound, or CT scans. These additional tools help confirm the diagnosis and rule out other potential causes of abdominal pain such as UTIs, ovarian cysts, or gastrointestinal disorders.

McBurney's sign is a valuable clinical tool for identifying appendicitis by pinpointing tenderness at McBurney's point in the right lower quadrant of the abdomen. While it is not definitive on its own, it plays a crucial role in the broader diagnostic process, helping healthcare providers make timely and accurate decisions to prevent complications such as appendix perforation or peritonitis. Its historical significance and continued use in clinical practice underscore its importance in the evaluation of abdominal pain.

2.3.2 Rovsing's sign

The sign is named after the Danish surgeon Niels Thorkild Rovsing, who first described it. The test involves palpating, or applying pressure, to the left lower quadrant of the abdomen, which is the area on the lower left side of the belly. When this pressure elicits pain in the right lower quadrant, the area on the lower right side of the abdomen, Rovsing's sign is considered positive. This phenomenon occurs because the pressure applied to the left side of the abdomen can transmit through the abdominal cavity and irritate the inflamed appendix on the right side. The pain referral to the right lower quadrant is a key indicator of appendicitis.

The underlying mechanism of Rovsing's sign is not entirely understood, but it is believed that the pressure causes movement or irritation of the inflamed appendix, leading to pain in its actual location. This sign is particularly useful because it helps differentiate appendicitis from other causes of abdominal pain such as gastrointestinal issues or gynecological conditions. However, Rovsing's sign is not definitive on its own and is typically used in conjunction with other clinical findings, such as rebound tenderness, McBurney's point tenderness, and laboratory or imaging tests like blood work, ultrasound, or CT scans.

In clinical practice, Rovsing's sign is one of several physical examination tools that healthcare providers use to assess the likelihood of appendicitis. Its presence, along with other symptoms like fever, nausea, vomiting, and localized right lower quadrant pain, can strengthen the suspicion of an inflamed appendix. Early diagnosis and treatment of appendicitis are crucial to prevent complications such as perforation, peritonitis, or abscess formation. Therefore, Rovsing's sign remains a valuable component of the diagnostic process for this common yet potentially serious condition.

2.3.3 Obturator sign

This sign is based on the anatomical relationship between the inflamed appendix and the obturator internus muscle, which is located in the pelvis and plays a role in the lateral rotation of the thigh. When the appendix becomes inflamed and irritates the obturator internus muscle, specific movements of the hip can elicit pain, which forms the basis of this diagnostic test.

To perform the obturator sign test, the patient is positioned supine, lying flat on their back on the examination table. The examiner then flexes the patient's right hip and knee to approximately 90. While maintaining this flexed position, the examiner internally rotates the hip by moving the patient's ankle laterally. This internal rotation stretches the obturator internus muscle. If the patient experiences pain in the hypogastric region, which is the lower central area of the abdomen, during this maneuver, the test is considered positive.

A positive obturator sign suggests that the inflamed appendix is likely in contact with or irritating the obturator internus muscle, indicating a pelvic location of the appendix. This finding can be particularly useful in cases where the presentation of appendicitis is atypical, as pelvic appendicitis may not always present with the classic symptoms of right lower quadrant pain.

2.3.4 The psoas sign

The psoas sign is a clinical test used to evaluate for acute appendicitis, particularly when the inflamed appendix is retrocecal in location, meaning it lies behind the cecum and in close proximity to the psoas major muscle. The psoas major muscle is a large muscle that runs from the lower spine through the pelvis and attaches to the femur, playing a key role in hip flexion and thigh movement. When the appendix is inflamed and irritates the psoas muscle, specific movements that stretch or contract this muscle can elicit pain, which forms the basis of the psoas sign.

To perform the psoas sign test, the patient is positioned supine, lying flat on their back on the examination table. The examiner then asks the patient to actively flex their right thigh at the hip, lifting their leg against resistance applied by the examiner's hand. Alternatively, the examiner may passively extend the patient's right hip while the patient lies on their left side. Both maneuvers involve stretching or engaging the psoas muscle. If the patient experiences pain in the right lower quadrant of the abdomen during these maneuvers, the test is considered positive.

A positive psoas sign suggests that the inflamed appendix is irritating the psoas major muscle, which is often the case when the appendix is retrocecal in position. This retrocecal location can alter the typical presentation of appendicitis, as the pain may not be localized to the classic McBurney's point (the area one-third of the distance from the ASIS to the umbilicus). Instead, the pain may be deeper or referred to the flank or back, making the psoas sign a valuable diagnostic clue in such cases.

The psoas sign is not specific to appendicitis and can also be seen in other conditions that involve irritation of the psoas muscle such as a psoas abscess, retroperitoneal inflammation, or certain musculoskeletal disorders. Therefore, like other clinical signs, the psoas sign must be interpreted in the context of the patient's overall clinical presentation, including their history, other physical examination findings, and diagnostic tests such as imaging or laboratory studies.

2.3.5 Interpretation of clinical signs

With advancements in imaging techniques such as CT and magnetic resonance imaging (MRI), traditional clinical signs of appendicitis are becoming less critical for decision-making in the emergency setting. These imaging modalities provide high-resolution, cross-sectional views of the appendix and surrounding structures, allowing for more accurate diagnosis, even in atypical cases or early disease stages. As a result, reliance on physical examination findings alone has diminished, though they still play a role in initial clinical assessment.

Pain in appendicitis can be exacerbated by even minor movements, such as coughing, sudden changes in position, or external vibrations, such as those experienced when driving over uneven roads. This phenomenon, often referred to as "bumps in the road" tenderness, underscores the peritoneal irritation associated with appendiceal inflammation.

During physical examination, a digital rectal exam is usually unremarkable unless the inflamed appendiceal tip extends into the pelvis. In such cases, deep tenderness may be elicited, or a mass may be palpated if a pelvic abscess has formed. The presence of a pelvic abscess may also lead to symptoms such as tenesmus, urinary urgency, or increased rectal discomfort.

Cervical motion tenderness, typically considered a hallmark of PID, can occasionally be observed in cases of appendicitis when inflammation spreads to adjacent pelvic structures. This overlap in clinical findings can lead to diagnostic uncertainty, particularly in female patients, where gynecologic conditions such as ovarian torsion, ectopic pregnancy, or endometriosis must also be considered in the differential diagnosis. In such cases, transvaginal ultrasound may be useful to rule out gynecologic pathology, while imaging with CT or MRI can confirm the presence of an inflamed appendix.

It is important to note that recent antibiotic therapy or concurrent systemic steroid use may suppress or mask the symptoms and signs of acute appendicitis. Diagnosis becomes more challenging when communication is limited such as in cases of language barriers, young children, individuals with dementia, mental health conditions, or learning disabilities. Additionally, age-related or disease-related changes in pain perception, such as those seen in diabetes, can reduce the ability to sense pain accurately. Consequently, diagnostic uncertainty is more common in obese individuals, children, immunocompromised patients, the elderly, and those on immunosuppressive therapy. In these special populations, a collateral history of decreased activity or reduced oral intake should raise clinical suspicion.

2.4 Laboratory and imaging studies

Laboratory studies serve as valuable adjuncts in the diagnosis of acute appendicitis, but they are not independently definitive. Their primary role is to support clinical evaluation and imaging rather than to establish the diagnosis on their own. While no single laboratory marker is both highly sensitive and specific for appendicitis, a combination of inflammatory markers can improve diagnostic accuracy, particularly in equivocal cases.

Numerous biomarkers have been investigated for their potential utility in diagnosing appendicitis, including WBC count, C-reactive protein (CRP), bilirubin, granulocyte colony-stimulating factor (G-CSF), fibrinogen, various interleukins, procalcitonin, the APPY1 test, and calprotectin. Among these, WBC count and CRP are most frequently used in clinical practice. Leukocytosis with a predominance of neutrophils is commonly seen in appendicitis, but its diagnostic utility is limited by its lack of specificity, as it can be elevated in many other inflammatory or infectious conditions. Additionally, its sensitivity is imperfect – one large study found that approximately 20% of patients with histologically confirmed appendicitis had a normal WBC count, underscoring the risk of false-negative results if laboratory findings are interpreted in isolation.

CRP, an acute-phase reactant, is another widely used inflammatory marker, but it is similarly unreliable when considered alone. While elevated CRP levels may indicate ongoing inflammation and can be helpful in distinguishing complicated from uncomplicated appendicitis, they lack specificity and can be elevated in various infectious and noninfectious conditions. Some studies suggest that combining WBC count and CRP measurement improves diagnostic accuracy, as a normal WBC and CRP together have a high negative predictive value for ruling out appendicitis.

Other emerging biomarkers, such as procalcitonin and calprotectin, have shown promise in research settings, particularly for identifying more severe or perforated cases of appendicitis. Elevated bilirubin levels have also been proposed as a potential indicator of appendiceal perforation, although their routine use in clinical practice remains limited. The APPY1 test, a newer point-of-care biomarker panel, has demonstrated some utility in pediatric populations for ruling out appendicitis, but further validation in broader patient cohorts is needed.

Ultimately, laboratory studies should be interpreted in the context of clinical findings and imaging results rather than being relied upon as standalone diagnostic tools. Their greatest value lies in refining clinical suspicion, guiding further investigation, and aiding in the risk stratification of patients presenting with suspected appendicitis.

Urinalysis is typically unremarkable in cases of acute appendicitis; however, mild abnormalities may occasionally be present due to the anatomical proximity of the inflamed appendix to the ureter or bladder. Trace amounts of leukocyte esterase, pyuria, or even microscopic hematuria can be detected, particularly when the appendix lies in a retrocecal or pelvic position, causing irritation of adjacent urinary structures.

Despite these findings, significant urinary abnormalities should prompt consideration of alternative diagnoses such as UTIs, nephrolithiasis, or gynecologic conditions in female patients.

In reproductive-age females, a urinary pregnancy test is a critical component of the diagnostic workup to exclude ectopic pregnancy, a potentially life-threatening condition that can present with overlapping symptoms including lower abdominal pain and peritoneal irritation. Failure to identify an ectopic pregnancy can lead to catastrophic consequences, making this test an essential step in the evaluation of women presenting with suspected appendicitis.

Hyperbilirubinemia has been observed in some cases of acute appendicitis, independent of underlying liver dysfunction or biliary obstruction. This phenomenon is thought to result from systemic inflammatory responses, bacterial cholestasis, or hepatic involvement due to bacterial translocation through the portal circulation. *Escherichia coli* endotoxins, for example, may contribute to transient hepatic dysfunction, leading to elevated bilirubin levels. Some studies have suggested that hyperbilirubinemia may be more common in cases of perforated appendicitis, raising interest in its potential role as a biomarker for disease severity. However, subsequent research has shown that bilirubin alone lacks sufficient sensitivity and specificity to reliably predict appendiceal perforation.

Given these limitations, while hyperbilirubinemia may raise suspicion for a more severe inflammatory process, it should not be used in isolation to guide clinical decision-making. Instead, it should be interpreted alongside other laboratory markers, imaging findings, and the overall clinical presentation to ensure accurate diagnosis and appropriate management.

The neutrophil-to-lymphocyte ratio increases with inflammation and has been proposed as a diagnostic marker with moderate accuracy. Elevated immature granulocytes indicate early bone marrow response to infection. However, a study by Jae-Sang Park et al. found that none of these biomarkers significantly improved diagnostic precision. The World Society of Emergency Surgery's Jerusalem Guidelines do not recommend routine use of any specific biomarker.

A range of imaging techniques assist in diagnosing appendicitis, with considerations including availability, radiation exposure, cost, execution time, and accuracy. Plain abdominal radiographs are generally unhelpful except to exclude perforation. A calcified fecalith in the right lower quadrant may suggest appendicitis but is present in only 5% of cases. Free air on imaging should raise suspicion of other hollow organ perforations.

Ultrasonography is considered a first-line imaging modality for diagnosing acute appendicitis, particularly in pediatric and pregnant patients, due to its noninvasive nature, lack of ionizing radiation, and widespread availability. When performed by experienced operators, ultrasound can effectively identify key features of an inflamed appendix, including increased diameter (typically >6 mm), wall thickening, lack of compressibility, and reduced peristaltic activity. Additionally, surrounding inflammatory changes, such as echogenic mesenteric fat or the presence of free fluid, can further support the diagnosis.

One of the primary advantages of ultrasonography is its real-time, dynamic assessment, allowing for targeted evaluation based on patient symptoms. However, its accuracy is highly dependent on the skill of the operator, patient body habitus, and appendix positioning. Retrocecal or deeply located appendices can be challenging to visualize, leading to nondiagnostic scans in up to 20–30% of cases. Sensitivity for detecting appendicitis ranges from 78% to 83%, while specificity is reported between 83% and 93%, making it a reliable but imperfect tool.

A study by Caruso et al. demonstrated a strong correlation between ultrasound findings and surgical confirmation, particularly in complicated cases such as perforated appendicitis or appendiceal abscess formation. In these scenarios, ultrasound can provide critical information regarding disease severity and guide further management decisions, including the need for immediate surgery versus conservative treatment with antibiotics and drainage.

Despite its utility, ultrasonography is often supplemented with CT or MRI when initial findings are inconclusive. In adult patients, CT remains the gold standard due to its superior sensitivity and specificity, while MRI is preferred in pregnant patients when further imaging is needed. Given its advantages and limitations, ultrasound remains a valuable first-line modality, particularly in specific patient populations, but should be interpreted within the broader clinical and diagnostic context.

CT scanning is the most accurate imaging modality for diagnosing acute appendicitis, offering high sensitivity and specificity that surpass other techniques. Its key advantages include objectivity, widespread availability, and consistent reliability regardless of patient body habitus, bowel gas interference, or the patient's ability to tolerate the examination due to pain. Unlike ultrasound, which is highly operator-dependent, CT provides reproducible, high-resolution images that allow for comprehensive evaluation of the appendix and surrounding structures.

A diseased appendix on CT typically appears enlarged, with an outer diameter exceeding 7 mm, a thickened and inflamed wall, and mural enhancement known as the "target sign" due to concentric rings of differing attenuation. Other findings supportive of appendicitis include periappendiceal fat stranding, free fluid, phlegmon, or abscess formation. If the appendix is not clearly visualized, the absence of surrounding inflammatory changes strongly suggests that appendicitis is unlikely. This feature enhances CT's utility in ruling out appendicitis, minimizing unnecessary surgeries and improving diagnostic confidence.

Routine CT use has significantly reduced the rate of negative appendectomies while also decreasing delays in diagnosis, particularly in cases with atypical presentations. Given concerns about radiation exposure, low-dose CT protocols have been investigated as an alternative to standard-dose CT. Multiple studies have demonstrated that low-dose CT maintains comparable diagnostic accuracy, with sensitivities and specificities approaching those of conventional CT. However, certain studies suggest that standard-dose CT may offer a 10% greater sensitivity in detecting alternative diagnoses, which is particularly relevant in elderly patients, where a broader range of pathologies must be considered. Additionally, standard-dose CT has been shown to have superior negative predictive value for identifying appendiceal perforation, which is critical for surgical planning and patient management.

Despite these advantages, CT should be used judiciously, particularly in pediatric and pregnant patients, where radiation exposure is a greater concern. In these populations, ultrasound remains the preferred first-line imaging modality, with MRI serving as a second-line option when additional imaging is needed. Overall, CT remains the gold standard for appendicitis diagnosis in adult patients, balancing accuracy, efficiency, and clinical utility in a wide range of presentations.

MRI is the preferred imaging modality for evaluating suspected appendicitis in pregnant patients, as it provides excellent soft tissue contrast without exposing the fetus to ionizing radiation. MRI has demonstrated high diagnostic accuracy, with reported sensitivity reaching 100% and specificity of approximately 98%, making it a reliable tool for confirming or ruling out appendicitis in this patient population. Unlike CT, which relies on ionizing radiation, MRI uses strong magnetic fields and radiofrequency pulses, making it a safer alternative, particularly in the second and third trimesters of pregnancy.

On MRI, an inflamed appendix typically appears enlarged, with an outer diameter exceeding 7 mm, luminal high-signal-intensity fluid on T2-weighted imaging, and periappendiceal fat stranding. In cases of complicated appendicitis, findings may include phlegmon or abscess formation. Importantly, MRI can detect early inflammatory changes that precede luminal dilation, such as periappendiceal edema, which may aid in diagnosing appendicitis at an earlier stage. Diffusion-weighted imaging has also been explored as an adjunct for improving diagnostic sensitivity by highlighting areas of restricted diffusion due to inflammation.

In addition to pregnant patients, MRI is increasingly utilized in pediatric patients when ultrasound findings are inconclusive. The ability to obtain detailed imaging without radiation exposure makes MRI particularly beneficial for children, where cumulative radiation doses from CT scans are a concern. However, MRI requires longer acquisition times and greater patient cooperation, which can be challenging in younger children or those experiencing severe pain.

A study by Moore et al. reported an MRI sensitivity of 96.5% and specificity of 96.1% for diagnosing appendicitis, further supporting its role as an effective alternative to CT in select patient populations. Despite its advantages, MRI is not as widely available as CT, and its use is often limited to tertiary care centers or cases where radiation avoidance is a priority. Nevertheless, as MRI technology continues to advance, its role in the diagnostic workup of appendicitis is likely to expand, particularly for vulnerable patient groups where minimizing radiation exposure is a key consideration.

While imaging provides objective and reproducible findings, it does not replace sound clinical judgment.

2.5 Scoring systems

Acute appendicitis remains a challenging diagnosis, and numerous attempts have been made to establish a reliable, evidence-based decision-making framework. However, no biomarker or scoring system currently achieves sufficient accuracy to predict acute appendicitis definitively. As a result, diagnosis continues to rely predominantly on patient history and physical examination. Nonetheless, the widespread availability and high diagnostic accuracy of CT and MRI have led many surgeons to incorporate these imaging modalities into their diagnostic approach. Scoring systems serve as a valuable tool for stratifying patients into low, moderate, and high-risk categories, aiding clinicians in determining the need for further testing, observation, or immediate surgical intervention.

The Alvarado score is particularly useful for ruling out appendicitis, with a reported sensitivity of 94–99%. Introduced in 1986, this system was designed as a simple and efficient tool for risk stratification, incorporating eight predictive factors derived from patient history, physical examination, and laboratory findings. These factors include right lower quadrant tenderness, leukocytosis, migratory pain, left shift of the leukocyte differential, fever, nausea and/or vomiting, anorexia, and rebound pain. Each criterion is assigned a specific point value, with the total score ranging from 1 to 10. A higher score correlates with an increased likelihood of appendicitis, aiding clinicians in decision-making regarding further diagnostic testing or surgical intervention.

A score below 4 suggests that appendicitis is unlikely, allowing clinicians to safely defer unnecessary imaging or surgery in favor of clinical observation or alternative diagnoses. Conversely, a score of 7 or higher is strongly suggestive of appendicitis and often warrants surgical intervention without additional imaging, especially in high-prevalence settings. Patients scoring in the intermediate range (4–6) present a diagnostic challenge, as they fall into a gray zone where neither immediate surgery nor complete exclusion of appendicitis is justified. To address this uncertainty, McKay and Shepherd validated the predictive value of the Alvarado score, recommending CT imaging for patients in this intermediate category to improve diagnostic accuracy before proceeding with operative management.

Despite its widespread use, the Alvarado score has notable limitations. Studies have shown that its accuracy varies among different patient populations. For example, it has been found to be less reliable in children, where clinical presentation can be atypical and symptoms may overlap with other common pediatric conditions. Similarly, in female patients, gynecologic conditions such as ovarian cyst rupture, PID, and ectopic pregnancy can mimic the symptoms of acute appendicitis, reducing the specificity of the score. Ohle et al. conducted a systematic review demonstrating that while the Alvarado score performs well in men, it tends to overpredict appendicitis in women and lacks sufficient discriminatory power in children.

Further studies have questioned the reliability of the Alvarado score as a stand-alone diagnostic tool. Apisarnthanarak et al. conducted a retrospective analysis comparing the Alvarado score with CT scans and found that nearly 50% of patients with confirmed acute appendicitis had low or equivocal scores, highlighting the risk of underdiagnosis if the score is used in isolation. As a result, many clinicians advocate for the use of imaging, particularly in equivocal cases, rather than relying solely on clinical scoring systems. Nonetheless, the Alvarado score remains a valuable adjunct in the initial assessment of suspected appendicitis, serving as a guide for further diagnostic steps and helping to reduce unnecessary imaging or operative procedures in low-risk patients.

The Appendicitis Inflammatory Response (AIR) score, introduced by Andersson in 2008, was developed to improve the diagnostic accuracy of clinical scoring systems for acute appendicitis, particularly by incorporating markers of inflammation. It has demonstrated superior predictive value compared to the Alvarado score, especially in assessing not only the presence of appendicitis but also its severity. This refined approach enhances clinical decision-making by reducing unnecessary surgeries and optimizing the use of advanced imaging.

Like the Alvarado score, the AIR score considers key clinical variables including right lower quadrant tenderness, rebound tenderness, fever, leukocytosis, and a left shift in the leukocyte differential. However, it introduces CRP as an additional biomarker of inflammation, which significantly enhances its predictive accuracy. Since CRP levels tend to rise in response to bacterial infection, their inclusion allows the AIR score to better differentiate appendicitis from other causes of abdominal pain.

The AIR score ranges from 0 to 12, with risk stratification into three distinct categories: low risk (<4), intermediate risk (5–8), and high risk (>8). Patients with low scores can often be managed conservatively, either through observation or alternative diagnoses, while those with high scores are more likely to require immediate surgical intervention. For patients in the intermediate-risk category, additional imaging, such as ultrasound or CT scan, is often recommended to clarify the diagnosis and prevent unnecessary surgery.

One of the key advantages of the AIR score is its applicability across different patient populations. Unlike the Alvarado score, which has been shown to be less reliable in children and women due to the influence of subjective symptoms, the AIR score relies more on objective clinical findings and laboratory values. This makes it particularly useful in pediatric cases, where history-taking may be limited, and in settings where clinical presentation is more variable. Additionally, research suggests that the AIR score may be more effective than the Alvarado score in predicting complicated appendicitis, providing surgeons with a better tool to anticipate the need for more aggressive management strategies.

Overall, while the AIR score is not yet universally adopted in clinical practice, its emphasis on inflammatory markers and objective data makes it a valuable complement to traditional clinical assessment. As further studies validate its use, it may become an increasingly integral part of decision-making algorithms for suspected appendicitis, helping to optimize patient care while minimizing unnecessary interventions.

In pediatric cases, the Pediatric Appendicitis Score (PAS) was developed as a specialized scoring system tailored to children, aiming to improve diagnostic accuracy for acute appendicitis in this population. The PAS incorporates clinical variables similar to those used in the Alvarado score but places greater emphasis on factors relevant to pediatric presentations such as fever, nausea, right lower quadrant tenderness, leukocytosis, and rebound pain. The score ranges from 0 to 10, with higher values indicating a greater likelihood of appendicitis.

Despite its targeted design, studies comparing the PAS and Alvarado score have found no significant difference in their predictive value. Both scoring systems exhibit similar sensitivity and specificity, yet neither demonstrates sufficient accuracy to be relied upon as a standalone diagnostic tool in pediatric patients. This limitation arises partly from the fact that children often present with nonspecific symptoms and a wide range of differential diagnoses including mesenteric lymphadenitis, gastroenteritis, and gynecologic conditions in adolescent females.

A prospective study evaluating the PAS and Alvarado score in children found that while both scores could help stratify risk levels, neither had adequate reliability to definitively confirm or exclude appendicitis without additional clinical assessment or imaging. In particular, both scoring systems tend to overestimate the likelihood of appendicitis, leading to potential overtreatment or unnecessary surgical interventions. Conversely, they may also fail to identify certain cases, especially in early or atypical presentations.

Given these findings, the PAS is best utilized as an adjunctive tool rather than a definitive diagnostic method. When applied in conjunction with imaging modalities such as ultrasound or MRI, it can aid in decision-making by helping clinicians determine which patients require further evaluation or observation. Additionally, serial scoring over time may provide valuable insights, as changes in score trends could indicate disease progression or resolution, further refining the clinical approach to pediatric appendicitis.

Ultimately, while the PAS offers a structured framework for assessing pediatric patients with suspected appendicitis, its limitations highlight the need for a comprehensive diagnostic strategy that integrates clinical judgment, laboratory findings, and imaging studies to achieve the most accurate and effective patient management.

The Adult Appendicitis Score (AAS) was developed as a comprehensive risk stratification tool to improve diagnostic accuracy in adult patients presenting with suspected acute appendicitis. Unlike earlier scoring systems, the AAS incorporates a broader range of clinical variables, including patient history, physical examination findings, and laboratory markers, allowing for a more nuanced assessment of appendicitis risk. The score stratifies patients into three categories: low, intermediate, and high risk, facilitating clinical decision-making by guiding the appropriate use of imaging and surgical intervention.

One of the primary advantages of the AAS is its reliability in reducing unnecessary surgeries while optimizing the use of advanced imaging techniques such as CT and MRI. A validation study conducted by Sammalkorpi et al. demonstrated that the AAS effectively classified nearly half of patients as high risk, while only 7% were categorized as low risk. These findings suggest that the AAS can aid clinicians in identifying patients who require immediate surgical evaluation versus those who may benefit from further imaging or observation.

A large-scale study encompassing 5,345 patients across 154 hospitals in the United Kingdom further validated the AAS, comparing its performance to other established scoring systems. The study found that the AAS was particularly effective in stratifying risk in female patients, outperforming alternative methods such as the Alvarado and AIR scores in this demographic. Conversely, in male patients, the AIR Score demonstrated greater accuracy, particularly in cases with atypical presentations. These findings underscore the importance of tailoring diagnostic approaches based on patient characteristics to maximize accuracy and minimize unnecessary interventions.

In clinical practice, the AAS serves as a valuable adjunct to imaging and laboratory findings, helping to streamline patient management while reducing diagnostic uncertainty. Its structured approach supports evidence-based decision-making, improving the balance between timely surgical intervention and the avoidance of negative appendectomies. Despite its strengths, the AAS – like other scoring systems – should not be used in isolation but rather as part of an integrated diagnostic strategy that includes imaging studies and clinical judgment to ensure optimal patient outcomes.

The RIPASA score was developed as a response to the need for a more accurate and culturally relevant diagnostic framework for acute appendicitis, particularly in Middle Eastern and Asian populations. Traditional scoring systems, such as the Alvarado score, were primarily designed based on Western patient cohorts, which may not fully capture the clinical nuances and variations in disease presentation observed in other regions. Recognizing this limitation, researchers sought to develop a scoring system that better reflects the demographic, epidemiological, and healthcare realities of these populations.

To achieve this, the RIPASA score incorporates a broader range of clinical parameters compared to conventional models. In addition to core diagnostic criteria such as right lower quadrant pain, fever, and leukocytosis, it includes demographic factors like age and gender, symptom duration, specific physical examination findings, and additional laboratory markers that enhance its predictive accuracy. By tailoring the scoring criteria to the distinct characteristics of Middle Eastern and Asian patients, the RIPASA score aims to provide a more precise risk stratification, improving early diagnosis and reducing unnecessary surgeries.

Since its introduction, the RIPASA score has undergone extensive validation across multiple clinical settings, consistently demonstrating superior diagnostic performance compared to traditional scoring systems, particularly in the target populations. Studies have shown that it offers higher sensitivity and specificity, leading to a significant reduction in the rate of negative appendectomies – an essential factor in minimizing surgical risks and healthcare costs. Furthermore, its adoption has been associated with improved patient outcomes by facilitating timely and appropriate surgical intervention while avoiding unnecessary procedures.

The development and success of the RIPASA score underscore the importance of region-specific diagnostic tools in modern medicine. Differences in disease prevalence, symptomatology, and healthcare infrastructure necessitate the adaptation of clinical decision-making frameworks to local contexts. By acknowledging these variations, the medical community can ensure more accurate diagnoses, optimize resource utilization, and ultimately provide more equitable and effective healthcare globally.

Despite their availability and potential benefits, scoring systems for conditions such as acute appendicitis are infrequently utilized in real-world clinical practice. This underuse may stem from factors such as time constraints, lack of familiarity, or perceived complexity in applying these tools during busy clinical workflows. However, these systems play a critical role in several aspects of patient care and clinical decision-making. For instance, they help clinicians identify patients who may benefit from advanced imaging, such as CT scans or ultrasounds, thereby reducing unnecessary radiation exposure or costs for low-risk individuals. They also provide a structured approach for reevaluating patients over time, particularly in cases where symptoms are ambiguous or evolving.

Beyond their immediate clinical utility, scoring systems contribute to broader healthcare goals. They offer an objective framework that standardizes risk assessments, which can be particularly valuable in cases of diagnostic uncertainty. This objectivity not only aids clinicians in making more informed decisions but also enhances comparability in research studies by ensuring consistent criteria are applied across different patient populations and settings. Furthermore, scoring systems can serve as legal safeguards by documenting that a standardized, evidence-based approach was followed in the diagnostic process, which can be crucial in cases of adverse outcomes or litigation.

While it is important to recognize that scoring systems alone cannot definitively diagnose acute appendicitis – as they are designed to complement, not replace, clinical judgment – they remain valuable adjuncts in optimizing patient management. By integrating these tools into practice, clinicians can improve diagnostic accuracy, streamline resource allocation, and ultimately enhance patient outcomes. Their role in bridging the gap between clinical expertise and evidence-based guidelines underscores their importance as part of a comprehensive approach to care.

2.6 Microbiology

The pathogenesis of acute appendicitis is primarily attributed to luminal obstruction, most commonly caused by either a fecalith or hypertrophic lymphoid tissue. This obstruction transforms the appendix, a narrow blind-ended pouch, into an environment conducive to bacterial proliferation, ultimately leading to inflammation. Historically, it was hypothesized that patients with acute appendicitis exhibited a higher prevalence of anaerobic bacteria in the appendix and ileum. However, advancements in technology, particularly gene sequencing, have revolutionized our ability to assess and quantitatively characterize the microbiome. These innovations have opened new avenues for research, suggesting that alterations in the appendiceal microbiome may play a pivotal role in the pathophysiology of acute appendicitis. Notably, studies have identified *Fusobacterium* as a dominant bacterium in patients with acute appendicitis, accompanied by a reduction in *Bacteroides* populations. These findings bolster the theory that appendicitis is fundamentally an inflammatory disease linked to shifts in immune function, potentially influenced by lifestyle changes associated with industrialization. This is further supported by epidemiological trends: while the incidence of appendicitis remains stable in industrialized nations, it is rising rapidly in newly industrialized countries, as detailed in the preceding chapter.

Microbiological analyses of inflamed appendices consistently reveal a polymicrobial environment composed of both aerobic and anaerobic bacteria, reflecting the diverse microbial community of the gastrointestinal tract. Among these, *E. coli*, and *Bacteroides* spp. are the most frequently isolated pathogens, emphasizing their central role in the pathogenesis of acute appendicitis. However, advances in molecular techniques, particularly 16S rRNA gene sequencing, have provided a more comprehensive view of the appendiceal microbiome, uncovering a far more complex bacterial ecosystem than previously recognized.

Recent sequencing studies have identified a broad range of bacterial phyla in patients with acute appendicitis, suggesting that microbial dysbiosis – rather than the mere presence of a single pathogen – may contribute to disease onset and progression. This evolving understanding of the appendiceal microbiota has shed light on the dynamic interplay between commensal and pathogenic bacteria in the development of inflammation. Notably, *Fusobacterium* spp. has emerged as a potentially significant contributor to appendicitis severity. Studies have demonstrated a strong association between *Fusobacterium* spp. and more severe forms of appendicitis, including gangrenous and perforated cases. The mechanisms underlying this correlation are not yet fully understood but may involve enhanced tissue invasion, immune evasion strategies, or the production of virulence factors that exacerbate local inflammation.

These findings not only deepen our understanding of the microbial contributions to appendicitis but also open new avenues for targeted therapeutic strategies. The potential role of specific bacterial species in modulating disease severity raises the possibility of future interventions, such as microbiome-based diagnostics, antimicrobial stewardship tailored to bacterial profiles, or even probiotic therapies aimed at restoring microbial balance. As research in this field continues to expand, a more refined and individualized approach to the management of acute appendicitis may emerge, optimizing patient outcomes while minimizing unnecessary surgical interventions.

A comparative microbiologic study by Baron and colleagues examined the differences between complicated and uncomplicated acute appendicitis. They reported similar frequencies of aerobic bacteria in both groups but noted a lower prevalence of *Enterococcus* spp., *Enterobacter cloacae*, and *Lactobacillus* spp. in complicated cases. Conversely, *Pseudomonas aeruginosa*, *Fusobacterium* spp., and *Clostridium perfringens* were more frequently isolated in complicated appendicitis. These observations have led to the hypothesis that microbial imbalances may contribute to the pathogenesis of complicated appendicitis. Similarly, Jackson et al. compared the microbiome of appendiceal lumens in patients with appendicitis and control cases, identifying significant differences in bacterial composition. Inflamed appendices showed increased levels of genera such as *Peptostreptococcus, Bilophila, Bulleidia, Fusobacterium, Mogibacterium, Aminobacterium, Proteus, Actinomyces, Aaerovorax, Anaerofilu,* and *Porphyromonas.* Furthermore, the microbiota of complicated appendicitis differed from that of uncomplicated cases, with elevated levels of *Bulleida, Fusibacterium, Prevotella, Porphyromonas,* and *Dialister.* These findings align with those of Garcia-Marın and colleagues, who reported a higher prevalence of gram-positive cocci, including *S. constellatus,* and anaerobic organisms in complicated appendicitis. Although increases in *P. aeruginosa, Streptococcus* spp., *Bacteroides fragilis,* and *Prevotella* spp. were observed, they did not reach statistical significance. Based on these results, the authors concluded that complicated and uncomplicated appendicitis should be regarded as distinct clinical entities. *E. coli* remains the most frequently isolated bacterium in appendicitis cases, demonstrating good susceptibility to amoxicillin-clavulanic acid and aminoglycosides, though slightly reduced sensitivity to ciprofloxacin. *Pseudomonas aeruginosa* is also isolated in a significant proportion of cases and poses a challenge due to its resistance to amoxicillin-clavulanic acid and ertapenem. Consequently, Obinwa et al. have recommended the inclusion of anti-pseudomonal antibiotics in the treatment of appendiceal peritonitis, particularly when local empiric antibiotic protocols lack coverage for *Pseudomonas.* Anaerobic bacteria are also commonly isolated, albeit with varying frequencies. The Surgical Infection Society's empiric antibiotic guidelines recommend agents such as amoxicillin-clavulanic acid, piperacillin-tazobactam, carbapenems, metronidazole plus aztreonam, cephalosporins, or aminoglycosides. However, routine peritoneal fluid cultures often yield low positive rates, especially in uncomplicated appendicitis. Additionally, these cultures typically isolate microorganisms with well-documented resistance profiles consistent with community-acquired intra-abdominal infections. Since culture results often take several days to become available – frequently after hospital discharge – their utility in guiding immediate treatment is limited. Current recommendations advocate for peritoneal fluid cultures in high-risk patients, such as those over 70 years of age, individuals with malignancies, significant cardiovascular, hepatic, or renal disease, hypoalbuminemia, generalized peritonitis, delayed initial treatment, or suspected infections with resistant pathogens. In contrast, routine peritoneal fluid cultures are not deemed necessary for lower-risk patients with community-acquired infections, as they are unlikely to influence antibiotic therapy decisions.

The evolving understanding of the appendiceal microbiome and its role in acute appendicitis highlights the importance of microbial imbalances in disease progression and severity. Historically, acute appendicitis was primarily attributed to luminal obstruction, often caused by fecaliths or lymphoid hyperplasia. However, recent research has shifted focus toward the intricate microbial ecosystem within the appendix, emphasizing its influence on both the onset and severity of inflammation. Advances in high-throughput gene sequencing, such as 16S rRNA sequencing and metagenomic analysis, have provided deeper insights into the microbial landscape of appendicitis. These studies have revealed distinct differences in bacterial composition between healthy individuals and those with appendicitis, identifying specific pathogens, including *Fusobacterium nucleatum*, *B. fragilis*, and *E. coli*, as potential contributors to disease pathogenesis. Moreover, shifts in microbial diversity and dysbiosis have been associated with varying clinical presentations, from uncomplicated inflammation to perforated appendicitis. Such findings not only enhance our comprehension of the disease but also inform more targeted approaches to antibiotic therapy and patient management. By identifying bacterial signatures linked to different disease severities, clinicians may refine antibiotic selection to improve treatment efficacy and reduce unnecessary surgical interventions. Additionally, the emerging role of the microbiome raises intriguing possibilities for noninvasive diagnostic biomarkers and preventive strategies, such as microbiota modulation through probiotics or selective antimicrobial therapies. As our understanding of the appendiceal microbiome continues to expand, further research may uncover novel therapeutic targets and refine current treatment paradigms, ultimately leading to more personalized and effective management strategies for patients with acute appendicitis.

2.7 Treatment

The treatment of acute appendicitis should be individualized based on the patient's clinical presentation, severity of disease, and overall health status. Appendectomy remains the gold standard for managing acute uncomplicated appendicitis, with both open and laparoscopic approaches being widely accepted. Scientific societies endorse these surgical methods as the primary treatment options. Initial management of acute appendicitis should include prompt fluid resuscitation, as patients often present with varying degrees of hypovolemia due to factors such as intra-abdominal infection, third-space fluid losses, reduced oral intake, and vomiting. Hypovolemia can lead to hypotension and impaired tissue perfusion, increasing the risk of complications, particularly in cases of perforation or diffuse peritonitis.

Intravenous fluid replacement, typically with isotonic crystalloids such as normal saline or Ringer's lactate, should be guided by clinical assessment of dehydration and tissue perfusion. Parameters such as heart rate, blood pressure, urine output, and serum lactate levels can help determine the adequacy of resuscitation. In hemodynamically unstable patients, more aggressive fluid administration may be necessary, alongside close monitoring for signs of fluid overload. Maintenance fluid requirements must also be considered, as oral intake is restricted in preparation for potential surgery. This is particularly relevant in pediatric and elderly patients, who may be more susceptible to dehydration and electrolyte imbalances. Electrolyte levels, including sodium, potassium, and chloride, should be regularly monitored, especially in patients with prolonged vomiting, diffuse peritonitis, or significant third-space losses. Correcting any imbalances is crucial, as abnormalities such as hypokalemia or metabolic acidosis can complicate recovery and increase perioperative risk.

Broad-spectrum intravenous antibiotics targeting gram-negative and anaerobic bacteria should be administered promptly once acute appendicitis is suspected, as early antimicrobial therapy reduces the risk of complications such as abscess formation, sepsis, and prolonged hospital stays. First-line regimens typically include a combination of a third-generation cephalosporin (e.g., ceftriaxone) or a beta-lactam/beta-lactamase inhibitor (e.g., piperacillin-tazobactam) along with metronidazole to ensure adequate anaerobic coverage. In cases of penicillin allergy or local resistance patterns necessitating alternative options, fluoroquinolones or carbapenems may be considered. This is especially critical in cases of perforated appendicitis or extensive peritoneal contamination, where bacterial translocation and a heightened inflammatory response can lead to significant systemic effects. In such scenarios, larger fluid volumes may be required to manage sepsis-induced vasodilation and third-space losses.

Clinical assessment of volume status can be challenging, particularly in young, otherwise healthy patients who may compensate for significant fluid losses without immediate changes in vital signs. Tachycardia and subtle signs of poor perfusion, such as cool extremities or delayed capillary refill, may be the earliest indicators of evolving shock. Similarly, altered mental status in children and the elderly can be subtle, manifesting as irritability, confusion, or lethargy rather than overt hemodynamic instability. Urine output, a valuable marker of perfusion, may not be immediately available to guide fluid management, especially in noncatheterized patients or those with delayed hospital presentation. In such cases, bedside ultrasound assessment of the inferior vena cava (IVC) diameter and collapsibility can provide additional guidance on fluid responsiveness. Close monitoring and early escalation of care, including vasopressor support if fluid resuscitation alone is insufficient, are crucial for optimizing outcomes in patients with severe appendicitis and sepsis.

The timing of surgery for acute appendicitis remains a topic of ongoing debate, as emerging evidence continues to refine management strategies. While some studies suggest that delays of less than 24 h do not significantly increase complication rates in uncomplicated cases, others have found that prolonged intervals between diagnosis and surgery may be associated with higher rates of perforation, postoperative ileus, and prolonged hospital stays. The risk of perforation increases with symptom duration, particularly beyond 48 h, making early intervention generally preferable. However, in select cases – such as stable patients with mild symptoms – short delays may allow for optimization of comorbidities, fluid resuscitation, and antibiotic administration without compromising outcomes.

Decisions regarding surgical timing should be made on a case-by-case basis, taking into account factors such as patient age, comorbidities, clinical stability, and the availability of surgical resources. Elderly patients, immunocompromised individuals, and those with significant medical conditions may benefit from preoperative optimization, whereas younger, otherwise healthy individuals may tolerate early surgery without additional risks. Additionally, patients presenting with perforated appendicitis and abscess formation may be candidates for initial nonoperative management with percutaneous drainage and antibiotics, followed by interval appendectomy in select cases.

Laparoscopic appendectomy has become the preferred approach for most patients due to its advantages over open surgery including reduced postoperative pain, shorter recovery time, and lower rates of wound infections. This approach is particularly beneficial for women of reproductive age, as it allows for better visualization of the pelvic region, aiding in the diagnosis of gynecologic conditions that may mimic appendicitis, such as ovarian cyst rupture or PID. In obese patients, laparoscopy may also offer improved outcomes by minimizing wound complications.

For uncomplicated cases, a single preoperative dose of broad-spectrum antibiotics is generally sufficient to reduce the risk of postoperative infections. Early postoperative measures, such as rapid advancement to oral intake and early ambulation, are encouraged to promote recovery and minimize complications such as venous thromboembolism or ileus. Most patients undergoing laparoscopic appendectomy can be discharged within 1–2 days postoperatively, with a return to normal activities within a week. However, patients with complicated appendicitis, including perforation or abscess, may require extended antibiotic therapy and longer hospitalization based on their clinical course.

In cases of perforated appendicitis or abscess formation, treatment requires a more aggressive and multidisciplinary approach to optimize patient outcomes and minimize complications. Patients often present with significant systemic inflammation, sepsis, and hemodynamic instability, necessitating extensive fluid resuscitation and electrolyte correction before surgery. Prompt intravenous administration of isotonic crystalloids, guided by hemodynamic parameters and urine output, is essential to restore intravascular volume and ensure adequate tissue perfusion.

Broad-spectrum antibiotics should be initiated immediately upon diagnosis to cover gram-negative and anaerobic bacteria, with regimens typically including a beta-lactam/beta-lactamase inhibitor (e.g., piperacillin-tazobactam) or a combination of a third-generation cephalosporin (e.g., ceftriaxone) and metronidazole. The optimal duration of postoperative antibiotic therapy remains a subject of debate, but current guidelines generally recommend continuation for 4–7 days, with duration guided by clinical improvement, inflammatory markers, and imaging findings. Intraoperative cultures of peritoneal lavage fluid can be useful for tailoring antibiotic therapy based on local resistance patterns, particularly in patients who do not respond adequately to empirical treatment.

In cases of perforated appendicitis or abscess formation, treatment requires a more aggressive and multidisciplinary approach to optimize patient outcomes and minimize complications. Patients often present with significant systemic inflammation, sepsis, and hemodynamic instability, necessitating extensive fluid resuscitation and electrolyte correction before surgery. Prompt intravenous administration of isotonic crystalloids, guided by hemodynamic parameters and urine output, is essential to restore intravascular volume and ensure adequate tissue perfusion.

Broad-spectrum antibiotics should be initiated immediately upon diagnosis to cover gram-negative and anaerobic bacteria, with regimens typically including a beta-lactam/beta-lactamase inhibitor (e.g., piperacillin-tazobactam) or a combination of a third-generation cephalosporin (e.g., ceftriaxone) and metronidazole. The optimal duration of postoperative antibiotic therapy remains a subject of debate, but current guidelines generally recommend continuation for 4–7 days, with duration guided by clinical improvement, inflammatory markers, and imaging findings. Intraoperative cultures of peritoneal lavage fluid can be useful for tailoring antibiotic therapy based on local resistance patterns, particularly in patients who do not respond adequately to empirical treatment. Abscess formation complicates approximately 10–20% of perforated appendicitis cases and represents a major source of morbidity. When an abscess is detected, percutaneous drainage is the preferred initial management strategy, offering a minimally invasive approach with high success rates. If percutaneous access is not feasible due to anatomical constraints, alternative drainage methods such as laparoscopic, transrectal, or transvaginal approaches may be considered. In select patients, particularly those with well-contained abscesses and mild symptoms, initial nonoperative management with antibiotics alone may be an option, followed by interval appendectomy after 6–8 weeks to reduce recurrence risk. Close postoperative monitoring and individualized management are essential to prevent complications and ensure optimal recovery in patients with complicated appendicitis.

Non-operative management, involving antibiotics and supportive care, has gained traction as an alternative to surgery for uncomplicated acute appendicitis. This approach is particularly appealing for patients at high surgical risk, such as those with significant comorbidities, advanced age, or contraindications to anesthesia. By avoiding surgery, nonoperative management eliminates the risks associated with anesthesia, postoperative complications, and surgical site infections (SSIs), which are concerns even in otherwise healthy individuals. However, conservative treatment carries a risk of failure, with approximately 20% of patients requiring readmission for recurrent symptoms within a year. This failure rate raises concerns about the long-term efficacy of antibiotic therapy, as some patients may experience recurrent episodes that ultimately necessitate appendectomy. While some studies suggest that nonoperative management is associated with fewer short-term complications, it has a higher failure rate compared to appendectomy, which remains the definitive treatment. The debate over nonoperative treatment is further complicated by the lack of long-term data on recurrence rates and the heterogeneity of existing studies. Variations in patient selection, antibiotic regimens, and follow-up duration contribute to the challenge of drawing definitive conclusions. For example, the NOTA study found a 14% recurrence rate in patients treated with antibiotics, all of whom were successfully managed without surgery upon recurrence, suggesting that repeated antibiotic therapy might be a viable option for select cases. Similarly, a randomized trial by Park et al. demonstrated that uncomplicated appendicitis could resolve spontaneously with supportive care alone, without antibiotics, suggesting that natural remission may play a role in recovery. Despite these findings, important questions remain unanswered. The potential for missed underlying pathology, such as occult neoplasms, in patients who do not undergo surgery is a concern that warrants further investigation. Additionally, patient preferences and the psychological burden of living with a potentially recurrent condition must be considered when discussing treatment options. Future research should focus on refining patient selection criteria, optimizing antibiotic regimens, and assessing long-term outcomes to better define the role of nonoperative management in clinical practice.

Stratifying appendicitis into complicated and uncomplicated cases has been proposed as a way to optimize treatment strategies and guide clinical decision-making. This classification helps identify patients who may benefit from nonoperative management while ensuring timely surgical intervention for those at higher risk of complications. Complicated appendicitis, defined by perforation, abscess formation, or symptoms persisting for more than 48 h, typically necessitates surgery due to the increased risk of sepsis, peritonitis, and prolonged morbidity. In these cases, a delayed or conservative approach could lead to worsening infection and adverse outcomes, making appendectomy the preferred treatment. However, for uncomplicated appendicitis – where there is no evidence of perforation or extensive inflammation – nonoperative management has emerged as a viable alternative to surgery. The APPAC study, a landmark trial comparing antibiotic therapy with immediate appendectomy, found that 73% of patients treated with antibiotics successfully avoided appendectomy within the first year. This finding supports the feasibility of conservative management in selected patients, particularly those seeking to avoid surgery and its associated risks. Moreover, follow-up data from the study suggest that even when recurrence occurs, subsequent treatment with antibiotics or surgery remains safe and effective.

Economic analyses further reinforce the potential benefits of nonoperative management, as it is associated with lower direct medical costs, shorter hospital stays, and faster recovery times compared to surgery. By reducing the need for operative resources and postoperative care, conservative treatment may also ease the burden on healthcare systems. However, these economic advantages must be balanced against the possibility of recurrence, which could lead to additional hospital visits and interventions. Despite promising results, further research is needed to refine patient selection criteria and determine the long-term outcomes of nonoperative treatment. Future studies should focus on optimizing antibiotic regimens, identifying predictive markers for treatment success, and assessing patient-reported outcomes to better inform shared decision-making between clinicians and patients.

For patients presenting with advanced inflammation or abscesses, non-operative management with antibiotics and percutaneous drainage is often preferred over immediate surgery. Interval appendectomy, traditionally performed weeks to months after the acute phase, is now being questioned due to the relatively low risk of recurrence (8% in pediatric patients over 8 years). However, the presence of an appendicolith on imaging may justify interval appendectomy, as it is associated with a higher risk of recurrence. The decision to perform interval appendectomy should consider factors such as patient age, comorbidities, and the potential for underlying neoplasms, particularly in adults over 40. Colonoscopy is recommended for adult patients after nonoperative management to rule out malignancies. Outpatient laparoscopic appendectomy protocols have been successfully implemented in some institutions, reducing hospital stays and healthcare costs for uncomplicated appendicitis. Studies have shown that this approach is safe, with low morbidity and readmission rates. Enhanced Recovery After Surgery protocols further support early discharge and ambulatory management, offering societal and economic benefits.

Amebic appendicitis, a rare but serious form of the disease caused by *Entamoeba histolytica*, requires a combination of surgical and antimicrobial treatment to achieve optimal outcomes. Unlike typical bacterial appendicitis, which may be managed nonoperatively in select cases, amebic appendicitis necessitates prompt appendectomy due to its aggressive nature and potential for complications such as perforation and peritonitis. Antimicrobial therapy, typically with metronidazole, is essential to eradicate the parasitic infection and prevent systemic dissemination. In some cases, additional antibiotics such as nitroimidazoles or luminal agents (e.g., paromomycin) may be required to eliminate intestinal colonization and reduce the risk of recurrence. Nonoperative management is not recommended due to the higher morbidity and mortality rates associated with delayed treatment. Delays in surgical intervention can lead to extensive tissue necrosis, abscess formation, and increased risk of systemic spread, particularly in immunocompromised patients. Early diagnosis and appropriate treatment are crucial to preventing severe complications and improving patient outcomes.

Postoperative complications following appendectomy can range from mild to severe and may significantly impact patient recovery. Common complications include intra-abdominal abscesses, which typically arise from inadequate drainage of infected fluid, wound infections due to bacterial contamination, and adhesive small bowel obstruction resulting from postoperative adhesions. While most of these complications can be managed with antibiotics, drainage procedures, or conservative measures, some may require surgical intervention. A rare but serious postoperative complication is stump appendicitis, which occurs when inflammation recurs in the residual appendix stump left after an incomplete appendectomy. This condition can mimic primary acute appendicitis, leading to diagnostic delays and potential complications such as perforation and peritonitis. Diagnosis is often challenging and typically requires imaging studies, such as ultrasound or contrast-enhanced CT scans, to identify the inflamed remnant. In some cases, surgical exploration may be necessary for definitive diagnosis. Treatment of stump appendicitis involves surgical resection of the remaining appendix tissue to prevent recurrence. While simple reexcision is often sufficient, more extensive procedures such as ileocecectomy or right hemicolectomy may be required in cases complicated by perforation, abscess formation, or suspected malignancy. Early recognition and prompt surgical management are crucial to preventing further morbidity and ensuring optimal patient outcomes.

Mortality from acute appendicitis is rare in developed countries due to widespread access to healthcare, advanced diagnostic tools, and timely surgical intervention. However, in low- and middle-income countries, appendicitis remains a significant cause of morbidity and mortality. Factors such as delays in seeking medical care, limited access to healthcare facilities, shortages of trained surgical personnel, and inadequate diagnostic resources contribute to poorer outcomes. In resource-limited settings, patients often present with advanced disease, including perforation and peritonitis, which significantly increase the risk of sepsis and death. Limited availability of antibiotics, anesthesia, and surgical equipment further exacerbates the challenges of managing complicated appendicitis. Additionally, cultural and socioeconomic factors, such as financial constraints and lack of awareness about the severity of symptoms, may delay hospital visits, leading to worse prognoses. Addressing these disparities requires a multifaceted approach. Strengthening healthcare infrastructure by increasing the availability of surgical services, particularly in rural and underserved areas, is crucial. Expanding surgical training programs and deploying mobile surgical teams can help bridge the gap in access to emergency care. Public health initiatives aimed at improving awareness of appendicitis symptoms and the importance of seeking timely medical attention are also essential. Furthermore, investment in telemedicine and diagnostic innovations, such as portable ultrasound devices, could facilitate earlier detection and referral of patients in remote regions. By improving healthcare accessibility, education, and timely surgical intervention, the burden of appendicitis-related mortality in LMICs can be significantly reduced, ensuring better outcomes for patients regardless of geographic location or socioeconomic status.

The management of acute appendicitis has evolved significantly, with a growing emphasis on tailored treatment strategies. While appendectomy remains the standard of care, nonoperative management and outpatient protocols offer viable alternatives for select patients. Advances in imaging, antibiotics, and minimally invasive techniques continue to improve outcomes, but further research is needed to optimize treatment algorithms and address disparities in care.

2.8 Surgical techniques

A variety of surgical techniques are available for appendectomy, with the laparoscopic approach now widely considered the standard of care. Minimally invasive techniques have been evolving since the 1990s, and as surgical technologies continue to advance, it is likely that additional approaches will be introduced in the future.

2.8.1 History of appendectomy

Ancient Egyptian medical papyri, such as the Ebers Papyrus (circa 1500 BCE), contain descriptions of abdominal pain, swelling, and digestive disturbances, yet there is no clear evidence that Egyptian physicians recognized the appendix as a distinct anatomical structure or understood its pathological significance. Their medical practice was based largely on a combination of empirical observations and supernatural beliefs, and surgical intervention for abdominal ailments was almost nonexistent due to the high risk of infection and the lack of effective anesthesia or antisepsis. Similarly, in ancient Greece, Hippocrates (460–370 BCE) wrote extensively about gastrointestinal disorders, including colic and intestinal obstructions, but his works do not explicitly reference the appendix or describe a condition resembling acute appendicitis. His understanding of disease was rooted in the humoral theory, which attributed illness to an imbalance of bodily fluids, and abdominal pain was often considered a consequence of dietary indiscretions or an excess of black bile.

In ancient Rome, Galen (129–216 CE) significantly advanced anatomical knowledge, yet his descriptions of the digestive system remained incomplete. Because human dissection was often restricted, Galen relied heavily on animal models, particularly primates, whose intestinal anatomy differs from that of humans. As a result, he did not provide an accurate description of the vermiform appendix, and his influence on medical thought persisted for over a thousand years, delaying a proper understanding of appendiceal pathology. During the medieval and early Renaissance periods, medical texts continued to discuss abdominal pain in vague terms, often attributing it to imbalances of the humors or supernatural causes. Physicians relied on bloodletting, purgatives, and dietary modifications rather than surgical intervention, as abdominal operations were associated with almost certain death due to infection and peritonitis. It was not until the rise of anatomical studies in the Renaissance that the appendix was properly identified, laying the groundwork for future advances in abdominal surgery.

During the Renaissance (fourteenth to seventeenth century), a profound transformation occurred in medical science, driven by renewed interest in human anatomy and direct observation through dissection. This period marked a departure from the rigid adherence to Galenic theories, which had dominated medical thought for over a millennium. One of the most significant figures in this revolution was Andreas Vesalius (1514–1564), a Flemish anatomist whose groundbreaking work *De Humani Corporis Fabrica* (1543) provided the most detailed and accurate description of human anatomy up to that time. Unlike his predecessors, Vesalius challenged Galen's reliance on animal dissections and insisted on direct human cadaveric study, which led to the first proper identification of the appendix as a distinct anatomical structure. However, despite its anatomical recognition, the function of the appendix remained unknown, and there was still no clear understanding of its role in disease. The Renaissance also witnessed a revival of surgical techniques, facilitated by improvements in knowledge of wound healing and infection control. Ambroise Paré (1510–1590), a French barber-surgeon, introduced innovations in surgical procedures, including ligature of blood vessels to control hemorrhage, which laid the foundation for safer surgical interventions. Although abdominal surgery was still largely avoided due to its high mortality rate, the period set the stage for later developments by emphasizing empirical observation and challenging traditional dogmas. The growing interest in postmortem examinations allowed physicians to encounter cases of inflamed or perforated appendices, though these were often misclassified as general peritonitis or intestinal obstruction. It was not until the eighteenth and nineteenth centuries, with the rise of pathology as a scientific discipline, that appendicitis was recognized as a distinct clinical entity, eventually leading to the development of appendectomy as a life-saving procedure.

Following the Renaissance, the medical field entered the early modern period, spanning the seventeenth and eighteenth centuries. This era was characterized by significant advances in anatomy, pathology, and surgical techniques, although abdominal surgery remained highly risky due to the persistent lack of effective anesthesia and antisepsis. The growing acceptance of human dissection allowed for more detailed descriptions of the appendix, and postmortem examinations frequently revealed cases of perforated appendicitis, although they were often misclassified as peritonitis or typhlitis, a term used at the time to describe inflammation of the cecum. Physicians began to recognize patterns of acute abdominal pain leading to fatal outcomes, but without a clear understanding of bacterial infection and sepsis, effective treatment remained elusive.

The eighteenth century saw the emergence of pathology as a distinct discipline, with figures such as Giovanni Battista Morgagni (1682–1771) emphasizing the importance of correlating symptoms with postmortem findings. Morgagni's seminal work *De Sedibus et Causis Morborum* (1761) described cases resembling appendicitis, linking clinical symptoms to anatomical pathology. However, surgical intervention was still not a viable treatment option, as opening the abdomen was almost always fatal. Instead, treatments relied on purgatives, bloodletting, and dietary restrictions, which were largely ineffective in preventing appendiceal rupture and subsequent peritonitis.

By the early nineteenth century, with the gradual acceptance of the germ theory of disease and the advent of better surgical techniques, physicians began to experiment with abdominal surgery. The first recorded successful appendectomy for acute appendicitis was performed in 1735 by French surgeon Claudius Amyand on an 11-year-old boy with an appendiceal abscess. However, this was an isolated case, and appendectomy did not become a standard procedure until the late nineteenth century, when antiseptic techniques and anesthesia made surgery safer. The growing understanding of abdominal pathology during this period laid the groundwork for the eventual widespread adoption of appendectomy as the definitive treatment for appendicitis.

2.8.2 Open appendectomy

The open appendectomy technique was first described by Charles McBurney in 1891 and has remained largely unchanged over time. McBurney, an American surgeon, detailed this approach as an effective means of treating acute appendicitis before the advent of minimally invasive techniques. Despite the widespread adoption of laparoscopic appendectomy in modern surgical practice, the open technique remains relevant, particularly in cases where laparoscopy is contraindicated, such as in patients with extensive intra-abdominal adhesions, severe peritonitis, or hemodynamic instability.

In a traditional open procedure, the patient is placed in the supine position on the operating table, ensuring optimal exposure of the lower right quadrant. The surgeon then selects between two primary incision techniques based on patient factors and surgeon preference. The oblique McBurney incision, typically about 3–5 cm in length, is made two-thirds of the way along an imaginary line drawn from the umbilicus to the ASIS (McBurney's point). This approach provides direct access to the appendix with minimal disruption to surrounding tissues. Alternatively, the linear Rockey-Davis incision, a transverse muscle-splitting approach, offers better cosmetic outcomes and may facilitate improved wound healing while maintaining adequate exposure.

The initial step of the operation involves gaining access to the peritoneal cavity and identifying the cecum, the proximal portion of the large intestine from which the appendix arises. Mobilization of the cecum through the incision allows the surgeon to expose the base of the appendix fully. A key anatomical landmark in this step is the presence of the teniae coli, three longitudinal bands of smooth muscle unique to the large intestine. These structures converge at the base of the appendix and help distinguish the cecum from the adjacent ileum, ensuring accurate identification of the appendix.

Once the cecum is adequately exposed, attention is turned to the mesoappendix, the fold of peritoneum containing the appendiceal artery, a branch of the ileocolic artery. Careful dissection of the mesoappendix is performed to isolate and ligate the appendiceal artery, preventing excessive bleeding. Hemostasis is crucial in this stage to reduce the risk of postoperative complications such as hematoma formation.

The next step is the ligation and transection of the appendix. A ligature is placed at the base of the appendix, securing it before it is transected. The appendiceal stump is then managed based on surgical preference and institutional protocol. Historically, surgeons favored stump inversion, believing that burying the stump within the cecal wall reduced the risk of stump leakage and fistula formation. This technique is achieved using a purse-string or Z-suture, which inverts the stump into the cecum. However, multiple studies have since demonstrated that there is no significant difference in postoperative complications between inverted and non-inverted stumps, leading many surgeons to forgo inversion in favor of a simpler, non-buried approach.

Following stump management, hemostasis is ensured through cauterization or additional ligation as needed. The peritoneal cavity may be irrigated, particularly in cases of perforated appendicitis or abscess formation, to reduce bacterial contamination. The final stage involves wound closure, which is performed in layers. The peritoneum, fascia, and muscle layers are approximated using absorbable sutures, while the skin is typically closed with either sutures, staples, or adhesive strips, depending on the surgeon's preference and the patient's healing characteristics. Proper wound closure minimizes the risk of dehiscence and SSIs.

While open appendectomy is gradually being replaced by laparoscopic techniques in many settings, it remains a valuable and essential procedure, particularly in resource-limited environments or emergency situations where laparoscopic equipment and expertise may not be readily available.

2.8.3 Laparoscopic appendectomy

Laparoscopic appendectomy was pioneered by German gynecologist Kurt Semm, who performed the first procedure in 1983. Semm, a pioneer in minimally invasive surgery, initially faced considerable skepticism from the surgical community, as laparoscopy was primarily used in gynecological procedures at the time. Many surgeons doubted the feasibility of performing an intra-abdominal general surgery procedure through small incisions. However, as advancements in laparoscopic instrumentation and techniques improved, laparoscopic appendectomy gained widespread acceptance due to its numerous advantages over the open approach, including reduced postoperative pain, shorter hospital stays, faster recovery, lower rates of wound infections, and improved cosmetic outcomes.

For a laparoscopic appendectomy, the patient is placed in the supine position with both arms secured at the sides, although the left arm is often tucked to optimize ergonomics and provide more space for the surgeon and assistant, who typically operate from the left side. A urinary catheter is inserted preoperatively to decompress the bladder and prevent accidental injury during trocar placement, especially in cases where a suprapubic port might be used. Additionally, intravenous access is preferably placed on the right side to avoid interference with the operating team and instrumentation.

The abdominal cavity is accessed through an incision at the umbilicus, usually using the closed (Veress needle) or open (Hasson) technique to establish pneumoperitoneum with carbon dioxide (CO_2). Insufflation to a pressure of 12–15 mmHg allows for adequate visualization of intra-abdominal structures. After creating the pneumoperitoneum, the primary trocar (typically a 10 mm trocar) is inserted at the umbilicus. Two additional trocars are placed under direct vision: one in the suprapubic or supraumbilical region and another in the left lower quadrant. Proper trocar placement follows a triangulated configuration, ensuring optimal instrument maneuverability and facilitating precise dissection.

Once trocars are placed, the initial step of the procedure involves identifying the cecum and appendix. This can sometimes be challenging, particularly in cases of appendiceal perforation, retrocecal positioning, or excessive adhesions due to previous inflammation or surgery. A grasper is used to elevate the appendix, exposing its base for further dissection. The mesoappendix, which contains the appendiceal artery (a branch of the ileocolic artery), must be carefully dissected and divided. This is typically done using an energy device such as a harmonic scalpel, monopolar electrocautery, bipolar energy, or metal clips.

The appendiceal base is then secured before transection. The most commonly used method is ligation with an endoloop, but in cases of severe inflammation, perforation, or friable tissue, a linear cutting stapler may be preferred. The stapler, though more costly, provides a more secure closure by excising a small portion of the cecum, reducing the risk of stump leakage and postoperative complications. Once transected, the resected appendix is placed into an endo-bag to prevent contamination and retrieved through the umbilical port.

Before completing the procedure, the abdominal cavity is irrigated with saline or antibiotic-containing solution, particularly in cases of perforated appendicitis or peritonitis, to reduce bacterial contamination and the risk of intra-abdominal abscess formation. Hemostasis is confirmed, ensuring no active bleeding before desufflating the abdomen. The trocar sites are then closed in layers, with fascial closure for 10 mm or larger trocar sites to prevent port-site hernia formation. Skin closure is typically done using sutures, staples, or adhesive dressings, optimizing cosmetic outcomes.

Among the various methods used for mesoappendix division, monopolar electrocautery remains the most cost-effective option, as it is widely available, quick, and rarely associated with complications such as thermal injury or conversion to open surgery. Several comparative studies have evaluated monopolar electrocautery, bipolar energy, endoclips, endoloops, and the harmonic scalpel, finding no significant differences in clinical outcomes, complication rates, or length of hospital stay. As a result, the choice of technique is largely dependent on surgeon preference, available resources, and cost considerations.

Laparoscopic appendectomy has now become the gold standard for appendicitis treatment in most institutions worldwide. Despite this, open appendectomy remains a viable option, particularly in resource-limited settings or in cases where laparoscopic surgery is contraindicated, such as extensive intra-abdominal adhesions, severe peritonitis, or hemodynamic instability.

2.8.4 Alternative minimally invasive techniques

In addition to conventional laparoscopic appendectomy, alternative approaches such as single incision laparoscopic surgery (SILS) and natural orifice transluminal endoscopic surgery (NOTES) have been explored, though they remain less commonly performed.

2.8.4.1 Single incision laparoscopic surgery (SILS)

SILS, first described in 1997 for laparoscopic cholecystectomy, represents an evolution of minimally invasive surgical techniques. Unlike conventional multiport laparoscopy, which requires multiple small incisions to accommodate separate trocars for the camera and instruments, SILS utilizes a single umbilical incision to access the peritoneal cavity. Through this single entry point, multiple specialized trocars or a single multi-channel port are inserted, allowing for the passage of laparoscopic instruments and the camera.

The primary advantage of SILS is its superior cosmetic outcome, as it eliminates visible scars outside the natural umbilical fold, leading to better patient satisfaction regarding postoperative aesthetics. Additionally, some studies suggest a reduction in postoperative pain and quicker recovery times due to fewer incisions. However, despite these potential benefits, SILS has not achieved widespread adoption in clinical practice. Several factors contribute to this limited acceptance, including the increased technical difficulty of the procedure, a longer operative time compared to standard laparoscopy, and higher associated costs. The constraints imposed by operating through a single port, such as reduced instrument triangulation and increased clashing of instruments, add to the complexity of the technique and require advanced surgical skills.

A meta-analysis of seven randomized controlled trials comparing SILS to conventional multiport laparoscopy found no significant differences in key clinical outcomes such as complication rates, length of hospital stay, or overall recovery. This lack of clear clinical superiority, combined with the challenges of implementation, has limited the widespread integration of SILS into routine surgical practice. Nevertheless,

SILS continues to be explored in various surgical fields, including appendectomy, colectomy, and gynecologic procedures, where further refinements in instrumentation and technique may enhance its feasibility and potential benefits.

2.8.4.2 Natural orifice transluminal endoscopic surgery (NOTES)

NOTES was first described in 2007 as a minimally invasive surgical technique that involves accessing the peritoneal cavity through a natural orifice, such as the stomach, vagina, or rectum, rather than through traditional laparoscopic incisions. By eliminating the need for external abdominal incisions, NOTES theoretically offers several advantages over conventional laparoscopy, including a reduced risk of wound infections, trocar site hernias, and postoperative neuropathic pain. Additionally, it has the potential to improve cosmesis and enhance recovery by minimizing surgical trauma to the abdominal wall.

Despite these theoretical benefits, widespread adoption of NOTES has been slow due to several limiting factors. The procedure is technically more challenging than standard laparoscopic surgery, requiring advanced endoscopic skills and specialized instruments that are not yet widely available. The increased complexity of the technique translates into longer operative times, a steeper learning curve for surgeons, and a higher overall cost, all of which contribute to its limited integration into routine surgical practice. Furthermore, NOTES carries its own set of potential complications, including the risk of visceral perforation, intra-abdominal infections, and difficulties in achieving adequate closure of the natural orifice used for entry.

A study analyzing the first 217 NOTES appendectomies provided important insights into the feasibility and safety profile of this approach. The study reported a median operative time of 96 min, which is longer than that of standard laparoscopic appendectomy. The median length of postoperative hospitalization was 3 days, and the overall complication rate was 6.5%. Among the complications observed, the most notable included abscess formation, intra-abdominal infections, postoperative bleeding, and gastric leaks in cases where transgastric access was utilized. These findings suggest that while NOTES is a viable alternative to conventional appendectomy in select cases, it has yet to demonstrate significant advantages that would justify its routine use over laparoscopic techniques.

An even more experimental approach, known as colonic endoluminal appendectomy, has been explored in a limited number of cases. This technique involves the removal of the appendix entirely via an endoscopic approach through the colon, eliminating the need for transabdominal access. In one particularly notable case, a patient with a history of transverse colostomy underwent a successful endoluminal appendectomy using a modified colonoscope. While this approach represents a remarkable technical achievement and a potential alternative for highly selected patients, it remains far from being a practical or widely applicable solution.

Overall, while NOTES and other innovative endoscopic approaches continue to be explored in surgical research, their current clinical utility remains limited. Traditional laparoscopic surgery continues to offer a well-established balance of safety, efficacy, and accessibility, making it the preferred standard for appendectomy and other minimally invasive procedures. Until significant technological advancements address the procedural challenges and cost concerns associated with NOTES, it is unlikely to replace existing laparoscopic techniques in routine surgical practice.

2.8.5 Open versus laparoscopic appendectomy: current trends and evidence

A 2013 multicenter study involving 95 centers and a total of 3,326 patients provided valuable insight into the evolving trends in appendectomy techniques within the United Kingdom. The study found that 66.3% of appendectomies were initiated laparoscopically, reflecting a significant shift toward minimally invasive surgery. This proportion has continued to increase over the years as laparoscopic techniques become more refined, and as technological advancements make the procedure more accessible and efficient. As a consequence of this shift, many surgical residents now complete their training with limited exposure to open appendectomy, a procedure that was once the standard approach for managing acute appendicitis.

Despite the declining prevalence of open appendectomy, proficiency in this technique remains an essential skill for surgeons, particularly in scenarios where laparoscopy is not feasible. In cases of extensive intra-abdominal adhesions from previous surgeries, severe inflammation, or hemodynamic instability, laparoscopic access may be technically challenging or even contraindicated. Furthermore, in resource-limited settings where laparoscopic equipment is unavailable or cost-prohibitive, open appendectomy remains a widely performed and effective alternative. Given these considerations, surgical training programs continue to emphasize the importance of maintaining competency in both laparoscopic and open techniques.

The debate between open and laparoscopic appendectomy has persisted for decades, with numerous studies evaluating the relative benefits and risks of each approach. Both techniques are considered safe and effective, with their respective advantages and limitations. A large-scale analysis of data from 222 hospitals participating in the American College of Surgeons National Surgical Quality Improvement Program (ACS NSQIP) provided strong evidence favoring laparoscopy in many cases. The study found that laparoscopic appendectomy was associated with lower rates of wound complications and deep SSIs, particularly in cases of uncomplicated appendicitis. The minimally invasive nature of the procedure reduces surgical trauma to the abdominal wall, leading to faster recovery times, reduced postoperative pain, and earlier return to normal activities.

However, in cases of complicated appendicitis – such as perforated appendicitis with abscess formation or diffuse peritonitis – the benefits of laparoscopic surgery must be carefully weighed against its potential risks. While laparoscopy was found to significantly reduce the incidence of wound infections in these patients, it carried a slightly increased risk of postoperative intra-abdominal abscess formation. This is thought to be related to the challenges of achieving complete peritoneal lavage and fluid drainage through minimally invasive techniques, as well as the potential for bacterial contamination during pneumoperitoneum creation and instrument exchange. As a result, some surgeons advocate for a selective approach, opting for open appendectomy in cases where they anticipate difficulties in laparoscopic peritoneal toilet and drainage.

Beyond its therapeutic advantages, laparoscopy also provides superior diagnostic capability, which can be particularly beneficial in cases of uncertain diagnosis. This advantage is especially relevant in female patients presenting with right lower quadrant pain, where differential diagnoses may include gynecologic conditions such as ovarian torsion, ruptured ovarian cysts, or PID. Additionally, laparoscopy allows for direct visualization of the entire abdominal cavity, making it a valuable tool when other pathologies such as IBD, cecal diverticulitis, or Meckel's diverticulum are suspected. The ability to both diagnose and treat intra-abdominal pathology in the same setting underscores the versatility of the laparoscopic approach.

While laparoscopic appendectomy has become the preferred technique in most cases due to its advantages in wound healing, postoperative recovery, and diagnostic utility, open appendectomy remains an indispensable skill for surgeons. Ongoing research and advancements in minimally invasive surgical techniques continue to refine the approach to appendicitis management, ensuring that surgical decisions are tailored to the specific needs of each patient.

2.8.6 Adjunctive considerations in appendectomy

Several adjunctive measures have been investigated to improve outcomes in appendectomy procedures, particularly in cases of complicated appendicitis. One such measure, the routine placement of surgical drains following appendectomy for perforated appendicitis, has been widely debated. Historically, drains were believed to reduce the risk of intra-abdominal abscess formation by facilitating the evacuation of infected fluid and preventing fluid collection. However, accumulating evidence now discourages their routine use. Multiple studies, including randomized controlled trials and meta-analyses, have shown that surgical drains do not significantly reduce the incidence of postoperative abscess formation. Instead, they may contribute to increased morbidity by serving as a potential nidus for infection, prolonging hospital stays, and increasing patient discomfort without offering substantial clinical benefits. Consequently, enhanced recovery protocols and modern surgical guidelines now recommend selective rather than routine drainage, reserving its use for specific cases where targeted drainage is deemed necessary based on intraoperative findings.

Another adjunctive measure that has been studied is prophylactic peritoneal irrigation during appendectomy. The rationale behind irrigation is to reduce the bacterial load within the peritoneal cavity, theoretically minimizing the risk of postoperative infections. However, studies comparing peritoneal irrigation with simple suction alone have found no significant difference in postoperative abscess rates in either adult or pediatric populations. Additionally, excessive irrigation may dilute and spread infectious material, potentially leading to unintended complications. As a result, current evidence supports the use of simple suction to remove purulent material and debris rather than routine peritoneal lavage. This approach aligns with modern principles of minimally invasive surgery, which prioritize efficiency and limit unnecessary interventions that do not confer clear benefits.

Conversely, one adjunct that has shown promising results is the use of wound ring protectors in open appendectomy. SSIs remain a concern, particularly in cases of perforated or gangrenous appendicitis where bacterial contamination is more pronounced. Wound ring protectors create a physical barrier between the contaminated intra-abdominal contents and the surgical incision, thereby reducing the likelihood of bacterial seeding. Meta-analyses have demonstrated that these devices can significantly lower the rate of SSIs, particularly in contaminated or dirty wounds, making them a valuable tool in optimizing postoperative outcomes for patients undergoing open appendectomy.

Despite the increasing predominance of laparoscopic appendectomy as the preferred surgical approach, proficiency in open appendectomy remains an essential skill for surgeons. Certain clinical scenarios, such as extensive adhesions from prior surgeries, hemodynamic instability, or limitations in laparoscopic equipment availability, may necessitate conversion to or primary use of open techniques. Continued advancements in minimally invasive technology, including robotic-assisted surgery and SILS, may further refine surgical practice in the future. However, the overarching goal remains the same: to optimize patient outcomes through safe, effective, and evidence-based surgical strategies that balance innovation with clinical pragmatism.

2.8.7 Robotic appendectomy

Robotic appendectomy represents a significant evolution in minimally invasive surgery, leveraging robotic-assisted platforms to optimize surgical precision, visualization, and ergonomic efficiency for the surgeon. Since its introduction in the early 2000s, this technique has become increasingly viable, particularly in complex cases where traditional laparoscopic surgery might be technically challenging. The procedure begins with the patient being placed in a supine position, followed by the establishment of pneumoperitoneum using a Veress needle or an open technique. Typically, four robotic ports are inserted strategically to allow optimal triangulation and access to the right lower quadrant, with an additional assistant port if needed. The surgical robot, such as the Da Vinci system, is then docked, and the surgeon operates from a console, manipulating robotic arms equipped with articulating instruments that provide superior dexterity and a 3D high-definition magnified view of the operative field.

The first critical step of robotic appendectomy is the identification of the cecum and appendix. This is facilitated by the robotic system's enhanced visualization, which allows for precise tissue differentiation, even in cases of severe inflammation or anatomical variations. Once the appendix is located, it is grasped and elevated, allowing for the careful dissection of the mesoappendix. The appendiceal artery is ligated using energy devices such as a robotic harmonic scalpel, bipolar vessel sealers, or endoscopic clips, minimizing blood loss. The base of the appendix is then secured, typically using endoloops, robotic suturing, or a stapler, depending on the surgeon's preference and intraoperative findings. The appendix is transected and retrieved using an endo-bag to prevent contamination of the peritoneal cavity. Peritoneal irrigation may be performed if purulent or fecal contamination is present, although studies suggest it may not significantly impact postoperative outcomes compared to simple suction.

Robotic appendectomy offers numerous advantages over conventional laparoscopic and open techniques. The enhanced dexterity of robotic instruments allows for precise movements that reduce the risk of iatrogenic injuries, particularly in cases of perforated appendicitis, dense adhesions, or anatomical anomalies. The ergonomic benefits of the robotic platform also alleviate surgeon fatigue, enabling greater control and efficiency during prolonged procedures. Furthermore, the improved visualization aids in distinguishing healthy from inflamed tissues, which is particularly beneficial in distinguishing complicated appendicitis from other intra-abdominal pathologies, reducing the likelihood of misdiagnosis. Studies have shown that robotic appendectomy results in comparable or even lower rates of postoperative complications such as wound infections, intra-abdominal abscesses, and ileus when compared to standard laparoscopy. The procedure also demonstrates potential benefits in terms of reduced postoperative pain and faster recovery, though these advantages remain under investigation. The robotic system also provides more stable camera control, eliminating the need for an assistant to hold and adjust the laparoscope. This reduces unintentional camera movements and improves procedural efficiency. In cases where suturing is necessary, such as with a complicated appendicitis requiring stump closure or intra-abdominal contamination, the robotic system allows for more precise and controlled suturing than standard laparoscopic techniques.

Despite its benefits, robotic appendectomy is not without its limitations. The most significant drawback is cost, as robotic surgery involves substantial initial investment, maintenance expenses, and longer operative times compared to standard laparoscopy. Additionally, robotic systems are not yet universally available, limiting access in many healthcare institutions. Training requirements for surgeons and operating room staff also pose a challenge, as proficiency in robotic techniques necessitates a

steep learning curve. Furthermore, some studies indicate that for routine appendectomy cases, the advantages of robotic assistance may not be significant enough to justify its higher costs, suggesting that its primary utility may lie in more complex scenarios such as appendiceal abscess, severe obesity, or cases requiring precise
suturing and dissection.

Looking ahead, the role of robotic appendectomy is expected to expand as advancements in robotic technology drive down costs and improve efficiency. Next-
generation robotic systems with smaller footprints, improved haptic feedback, and
automated surgical assistance may enhance the feasibility and adoption of robotic appendectomy in a wider range of healthcare settings. Ongoing studies continue to assess the long-term benefits of robotic surgery in appendiceal pathology, with an emphasis on patient outcomes, cost-effectiveness, and learning curve optimization.
While laparoscopic appendectomy remains the gold standard for most cases today,
robotic-assisted techniques are likely to play an increasing role in complex and high-
risk patients, shaping the future landscape of minimally invasive appendiceal
surgery.

2.9 Surgical circumstances and special populations

Certain clinical scenarios involve specific patient populations or circumstances that
warrant special considerations. One of the ongoing debates in appendiceal surgery is
whether to remove a grossly normal appendix encountered during an operation performed for suspected appendicitis. Before making this decision, a thorough evaluation
of the abdominal and pelvic organs should be undertaken to rule out alternative
causes of the patient's symptoms. This is particularly facilitated when a laparoscopic
approach is utilized, as it provides a superior view of intra-abdominal structures. Any
intra-abdominal fluid should be analyzed in terms of volume, color, and biochemical
composition to gain insights into the underlying pathology. Additionally, the terminal
60 centimeters of the ileum should be carefully inspected to identify a Meckel's diverticulum or early signs of IBD. Indeed, initial presentations of undiagnosed Crohn's disease can manifest as terminal ileitis, mimicking acute appendicitis. A detailed examination of the ileal mesentery may reveal enlarged lymph nodes indicative of
mesenteric adenitis, further complicating the differential diagnosis.

If all other potential causes of right lower quadrant pain have been excluded, prophylactic removal of the appendix may be advisable for several reasons. First, many
conditions that present with right lower quadrant pain have a tendency to recur, and
an appendectomy eliminates one potential diagnostic uncertainty in future episodes.
Furthermore, a form of appendiceal pathology known as neurogenic appendicitis,
previously discussed, may cause significant abdominal pain despite the absence of
overt macroscopic or histopathologic abnormalities. Additionally, certain appendiceal
abnormalities not apparent during surgery may later be identified upon histopatho-

logic examination, including conditions such as low-grade appendiceal neoplasms or chronic inflammatory changes. Some patients experience recurrent episodes of right lower quadrant pain suggestive of intermittent appendiceal inflammation. Since acute appendicitis is known to occasionally resolve spontaneously, it is plausible that some individuals suffer from recurrent bouts of subclinical inflammation, which may later be confirmed by histopathology as chronic appendicitis. However, when radiologic findings, such as appendiceal wall thickening, are absent, other potential etiologies should be thoroughly investigated before proceeding with an appendectomy.

Incidental appendectomy, defined as the removal of the appendix during an unrelated abdominal surgery, was once routinely performed, particularly in younger patients, to prevent future episodes of appendicitis and avoid reoperation. However, this practice has been subject to increasing scrutiny. It is not without risks, including postoperative complications such as infection, bowel injury, or adhesions, and its benefits have been challenged by the evolving understanding of the appendix as an immunologically active organ rather than a vestigial remnant. Additionally, studies have demonstrated that incidental appendectomy is not cost-effective, further dissuading its routine implementation.

2.9.1 Special populations

2.9.1.1 Pregnant patients

Pregnant individuals represent a unique patient population requiring careful clinical assessment. Appendicitis is the most common nonobstetric surgical emergency during pregnancy and one of the most frequent indications for surgery in pregnant women. The incidence of acute appendicitis during pregnancy has been estimated between 1 in 1,250 and 1 in 1,500 pregnancies. Interestingly, research by Zingone et al. suggests that the risk of acute appendicitis is actually lower during pregnancy, particularly in the third trimester, which may be attributable to both biological and behavioral factors. One hypothesis posits that pregnancy induces immunologic alterations, shifting the balance toward a predominance of T-helper-2 cells over T-helper-1 cells, which could theoretically mitigate inflammatory conditions such as appendicitis and IBD. Additionally, smoking, a known risk factor for appendicitis due to its proinflammatory effects, is often reduced or discontinued during pregnancy, potentially contributing to the observed decline in appendicitis rates.

Diagnosing appendicitis in pregnancy is challenging due to anatomical and physiological changes that obscure classical clinical signs. The typical symptoms of appendicitis, already variable in the general population, are even less reliable during pregnancy, with classical presentations occurring in only 50–60% of cases. Nausea and vomiting, common early symptoms of appendicitis, are even less specific during pregnancy, while fever may be absent or lower than expected. The enlarging uterus displaces abdominal structures, making localization of pain more difficult and altering the position of the appendix, which can migrate superiorly as pregnancy progresses. Additionally, a common differential diagnosis in the second trimester is "round ligament pain," which results from the stretching of the suspensory ligaments of the uterus and can mimic appendicitis.

Laboratory markers are also less reliable in pregnancy. Mild leukocytosis and elevated CRP levels are commonly seen in pregnant women and do not necessarily indicate an ongoing inflammatory process. Given the overlapping clinical features with obstetric conditions, gynecologic evaluation should be an integral part of the assessment. The rate of negative appendectomy (removal of a noninflamed appendix) in pregnant women is particularly high, reaching up to 50% in some studies. Unfortunately, both acute appendicitis and negative appendectomy have detrimental effects on pregnancy, with risks of preterm labor (11%) and fetal loss (6%) in confirmed appendicitis cases, while negative appendectomy is still associated with a 10% risk of preterm labor and a 4% risk of fetal loss.

Given these concerns, improving diagnostic accuracy is essential. As pregnancy advances, the accuracy of diagnosis declines due to increasing anatomical distortion, leading to higher risks of appendiceal perforation and associated complications. Imaging plays a critical role in improving diagnostic precision. Ultrasound is typically the first-line imaging modality, but its sensitivity decreases as the uterus enlarges. MRI without contrast has emerged as the preferred imaging technique for suspected appendicitis in pregnant women due to its excellent diagnostic accuracy and safety. Routine use of MRI has been shown to reduce the negative appendectomy rate by 47% and is considered cost-effective. When MRI is unavailable, a limited CT scan can be performed, as the radiation dose used is generally below the threshold for fetal harm, especially in the second and third trimesters when organogenesis is complete.

There is an ongoing debate about whether an open or laparoscopic approach should be used for appendectomy in pregnant patients. Some studies have suggested higher fetal loss rates with laparoscopic appendectomy compared to open surgery, while others have reported superior outcomes with laparoscopy. Although pneumoperitoneum raises concerns about increased intra-abdominal pressure and its potential effects on respiratory physiology, the Society of American Gastrointestinal Endoscopic Surgeons now fully supports the use of laparoscopy during all trimesters of pregnancy, considering it safe and feasible.

2.9.1.2 Obese patients

Laparoscopic appendectomy offers distinct advantages in obese patients, addressing many of the technical challenges associated with open surgery in this population. In obese individuals, the presence of a thick subcutaneous fat layer can make open incisions more difficult to manage, increasing the risk of wound complications including infections, delayed healing, and incisional hernias. Additionally, larger incisions may contribute to increased postoperative pain and longer recovery times. By contrast, laparoscopy minimizes the need for large abdominal incisions, allowing for a less invasive approach that is particularly beneficial in patients with high body mass index.

Multiple studies analyzing outcomes in both pediatric and adult obese patients undergoing laparoscopic appendectomy have reinforced the safety and efficacy of this approach. Contrary to early concerns that obesity might independently increase the risk of postoperative complications, research has consistently shown that laparoscopic appendectomy in obese patients is associated with favorable outcomes. In particular, studies have demonstrated that laparoscopy in obese individuals is linked to reduced mortality, lower rates of wound infections, and shorter hospital stays compared to open appendectomy. The decreased incidence of wound infections is especially significant, given that obesity is a well-established risk factor for SSIs in open procedures due to impaired tissue oxygenation, increased bacterial colonization, and challenges in postoperative wound care.

Moreover, laparoscopic surgery offers additional benefits in obese patients beyond just reducing wound-related complications. The enhanced visualization provided by laparoscopy allows for precise dissection and improved access to the appendix, even in patients with significant visceral fat. The pneumoperitoneum created during laparoscopy also facilitates exposure of the surgical field, aiding in the identification of adjacent structures and reducing the likelihood of inadvertent injury. These factors contribute to lower overall complication rates and better surgical efficiency in experienced hands.

As the prevalence of obesity continues to rise globally, the role of minimally invasive techniques in general surgery is becoming increasingly important. While open appendectomy remains a viable option in select cases, the overwhelming evidence supports laparoscopy as the preferred approach for obese patients. The combination of reduced surgical trauma, lower infection risk, and faster postoperative recovery underscores its superiority, making it the standard of care in most centers worldwide.

2.9.1.3 Elderly patients

Although appendicitis is most commonly diagnosed in young adults, it remains a significant clinical concern in the elderly population. In older adults, the diagnosis of acute appendicitis can be particularly challenging due to atypical presentations and a broader differential diagnosis that includes serious conditions such as colorectal malignancies, ischemic bowel disease, and diverticulitis. The presence of age-related immunologic senescence can further obscure clinical findings, leading to a blunted inflammatory response and an absence of classic symptoms such as localized right lower quadrant pain and leukocytosis. As a result, appendicitis in elderly patients is more likely to be diagnosed at a later stage, increasing the risk of complications such as appendiceal perforation, abscess formation, and generalized peritonitis.

Delayed diagnosis in this population is associated with significantly worse outcomes compared to younger patients. Studies have shown that elderly individuals presenting with appendicitis have a higher likelihood of complicated disease, necessitating more extensive surgical intervention and prolonged recovery periods. Furthermore, the presence of multiple comorbidities, including cardiovascular disease, diabetes mellitus, and chronic kidney disease, increases the risk of postoperative morbidity and mortality. These factors underscore the importance of timely and accurate diagnosis in elderly patients with suspected appendicitis.

CT imaging plays a crucial role in the evaluation of acute appendicitis in older adults. Given the broader range of possible diagnoses and the often subtle or atypical clinical presentation, CT scanning provides valuable information that aids in both confirming the diagnosis and ruling out alternative pathologies. High-resolution CT imaging has demonstrated excellent sensitivity and specificity in detecting appendicitis, allowing for earlier intervention and improved patient outcomes.

When surgical management is indicated, laparoscopic appendectomy has been shown to be both safe and beneficial in elderly patients. Compared to open appendectomy, laparoscopy is associated with reduced postoperative complications, including lower rates of wound infections, shorter hospital stays, and faster recovery times. Additionally, laparoscopic surgery results in lower postoperative mortality rates, likely due to the reduced surgical trauma, improved pain control, and earlier mobilization that minimally invasive techniques provide. The enhanced visualization offered by laparoscopy is particularly advantageous in elderly patients, allowing for thorough intra-abdominal assessment and facilitating the identification of any concurrent pathology, such as malignancy or diverticular disease.

Despite these advantages, patient selection remains critical, as some elderly individuals with severe comorbidities or hemodynamic instability may not be ideal candidates for laparoscopy. In such cases, an individualized approach should be taken, weighing the risks and benefits of minimally invasive versus open surgical techniques. Regardless of the chosen approach, optimizing perioperative care – including early diagnosis, appropriate fluid resuscitation, and meticulous postoperative monitoring – is essential to improving outcomes in this vulnerable patient population.

2.9.1.4 Immunocompromised patients

In immunocompromised patients, including those receiving chronic immunosuppressive therapy, undergoing chemotherapy, or living with conditions such as HIV/AIDS, the clinical presentation of appendicitis can be atypical and insidious. Due to an impaired inflammatory response, these patients may not exhibit classic signs such as localized right lower quadrant pain, fever, or leukocytosis. Instead, symptoms may be vague or nonspecific, such as mild abdominal discomfort, anorexia, or low-grade fever, leading to delays in diagnosis and an increased risk of complications. Given these diagnostic challenges, a high index of suspicion is required, particularly in patients who present with unexplained abdominal symptoms. Early imaging with CT or ultrasound can be invaluable in confirming the diagnosis and guiding timely surgical intervention.

Among pediatric populations, children with cystic fibrosis (CF) represent a unique subset of patients with distinct appendiceal pathology. While the overall incidence of acute appendicitis is lower in children with CF compared to the general population, those who do develop appendicitis face a significantly higher risk of perforation. This increased risk is likely due to both the delayed recognition of symptoms and the altered pathophysiology associated with CF. Thick, inspissated mucus within the gastrointestinal tract can contribute to luminal obstruction and atypical presentations, making early detection challenging. Furthermore, chronic gastrointestinal symptoms common in CF, such as abdominal pain and constipation, may mask or mimic appendicitis, leading to further diagnostic uncertainty.

A key differential diagnosis in CF patients with suspected appendicitis is distal intestinal obstruction syndrome (DIOS). DIOS results from the accumulation of thickened intestinal contents in the distal ileum and cecum, leading to partial or complete obstruction. Its presentation often overlaps with appendicitis, including right lower quadrant pain, nausea, and vomiting. However, DIOS is typically managed conservatively with aggressive hydration, osmotic laxatives, and sometimes enemas, whereas appendicitis requires surgical intervention. Differentiating between these conditions is critical to avoid unnecessary surgery or inappropriate medical management. CT imaging can be particularly useful in distinguishing DIOS from appendicitis by revealing characteristic findings such as dilated bowel loops with inspissated stool in the ileocecal region.

Given these complexities, the management of appendicitis in immunocompromised and CF patients requires a tailored approach. Prompt imaging, close clinical monitoring, and a multidisciplinary team involving surgeons, infectious disease specialists, and gastroenterologists are essential to optimizing outcomes. In surgical cases, a laparoscopic approach is generally preferred due to its reduced risk of wound infections and shorter recovery time, although individualized considerations should be made based on the patient's overall health status and surgical risk factors.

2.9.2 Complications of appendectomy

Appendectomy, whether performed via open, laparoscopic, or robotic techniques, is generally a safe and effective procedure for treating acute appendicitis. However, like any surgical intervention, it carries a risk of complications, ranging from mild, self-limiting issues to severe, life-threatening conditions requiring urgent intervention. These complications can be categorized into intraoperative and postoperative issues.

Among intraoperative complications, bleeding is a concern, especially if the appendicular artery, the ileocolic artery, or other mesenteric vessels are inadvertently injured. While uncommon, hemorrhage can necessitate conversion to an open procedure for adequate hemostasis. Another potential issue is bowel injury, which may occur due to iatrogenic trauma to the small intestine, cecum, or colon. This is particularly risky in cases of perforated appendicitis with extensive inflammation and adhesions. Laparoscopic and robotic approaches, despite their advantages, can increase the risk of bowel injury due to the lack of tactile feedback. Urinary tract injury is another possible complication, especially involving the right ureter in cases of retrocecal appendicitis or severe inflammation. If unnoticed during surgery, ureteral injuries can present later with flank pain, hematuria, or urinary leakage.

In some instances, a laparoscopic or robotic appendectomy may need to be converted to an open procedure due to severe adhesions, uncontrolled bleeding, extensive abscess formation, or failure to safely identify critical structures. While conversion itself is not a complication, it increases operative time and may lead to higher postoperative morbidity.

Postoperative complications are more common and can significantly impact recovery. One of the most frequent issues is SSI, which can be superficial or deep. Superficial infections involve the skin and subcutaneous tissue, presenting with redness, swelling, and purulent discharge, whereas deep infections may involve the muscle and fascia, requiring drainage and antibiotic therapy. The risk of infection is notably higher in cases of perforated appendicitis.

Beyond localized infections, intra-abdominal abscess formation is a serious complication, particularly following perforated or gangrenous appendicitis. These abscesses often develop within the pelvis, subphrenic space, or peritoneal cavity and present with fever, localized pain, and systemic signs of infection. Management may involve percutaneous drainage under radiologic guidance or, in severe cases, reoperation.

Postoperative ileus, a transient impairment of bowel motility, can occur after appendectomy, leading to abdominal distension, nausea, vomiting, and failure to pass flatus or stool. This condition typically resolves within a few days with supportive care, including nasogastric decompression and fluid management. However, a prolonged ileus may indicate a more serious underlying complication, such as infection or bowel injury.

Another potential consequence of surgery is adhesion formation, which may lead to bowel obstruction. This risk is particularly high after open appendectomy, though it can also occur following laparoscopic procedures. Patients may present weeks or even years later with cramping abdominal pain, nausea, and vomiting, sometimes necessitating surgical intervention for adhesiolysis.

A rare but significant complication is stump appendicitis, which occurs when a residual portion of the appendiceal stump becomes inflamed. This condition arises due to incomplete removal of the appendix and leads to recurrent symptoms similar to acute appendicitis. Diagnosis is often delayed, and definitive treatment requires reoperation to excise the remaining stump.

Fecal fistula is another possible complication, particularly when the cecum or terminal ileum is inadvertently injured during surgery. This leads to a fistulous connection between the bowel and the peritoneal cavity or the skin, presenting with persistent abdominal pain, discharge of enteric contents, and signs of sepsis. Management may involve bowel rest, parenteral nutrition, and, in some cases, surgical repair.

Port-site hernias can develop after laparoscopic appendectomy, especially if large trocar sites are not properly closed. These hernias may present with localized bulging and discomfort at the incision site and, in severe cases, can lead to bowel obstruction or strangulation, requiring surgical repair.

Venous thromboembolism, including deep vein thrombosis (DVT) and pulmonary embolism, is another concern, particularly in patients with prolonged hospitalization or limited mobility. Prophylactic anticoagulation and early ambulation play a crucial role in reducing this risk.

Some patients experience chronic post-appendectomy pain syndrome, a condition characterized by persistent abdominal pain without a clear underlying cause. This syndrome is sometimes linked to nerve entrapment or adhesions and can significantly impact quality of life, requiring further evaluation and symptomatic management.

While the mortality risk associated with appendectomy is generally low, typically below 1%, it increases in elderly patients, those with severe comorbidities, and in cases of delayed diagnosis of perforated appendicitis with sepsis.

While appendectomy is a routine surgical procedure with a generally favorable outcome, complications can still arise. Awareness of potential intraoperative and postoperative issues allows for timely recognition and appropriate management. Advances in minimally invasive techniques, including robotic surgery, may help reduce some of these risks, but careful patient selection, meticulous surgical technique, and prompt postoperative care remain essential in optimizing outcomes.

2.9.3 Postoperative care and recovery after appendectomy

Postoperative care following an appendectomy is crucial for ensuring a smooth recovery, minimizing complications, and facilitating a return to normal activities. Recovery varies depending on whether the procedure was performed as an open, laparoscopic, or robotic surgery and on the presence of complications such as perforation, peritonitis, or abscess formation.

2.9.3.1 Immediate postoperative period
After surgery, patients are typically monitored in the postanesthesia care unit until they recover from anesthesia. Vital signs, pain levels, and overall stability are assessed before transfer to a hospital ward or, in the case of uncomplicated laparoscopic appendectomy, discharge home the same day. Pain management is initiated early,

often with a combination of nonopioid analgesics such as acetaminophen and NSAIDs, while opioids are reserved for severe pain.

Intravenous fluids are maintained until the patient is able to tolerate oral intake. Nausea and vomiting, common in the immediate postoperative period, are managed with antiemetics like ondansetron. Patients are encouraged to start with clear liquids and progress to a normal diet as tolerated. Early mobilization is encouraged to prevent venous thromboembolism, improve bowel function, and reduce the risk of postoperative ileus.

2.9.3.2 Hospital stay and discharge criteria

The length of hospital stay depends on the surgical approach and whether complications are present. Patients undergoing uncomplicated laparoscopic appendectomy may be discharged within 24–48 h, while those with complicated appendicitis, intra-abdominal abscesses, or sepsis may require several days of inpatient monitoring. Discharge criteria include stable vital signs, adequate pain control with oral medications, tolerance of oral intake, absence of severe nausea or vomiting, and ability to ambulate independently.

For cases of perforated appendicitis or intra-abdominal infection, intravenous antibiotics may be continued postoperatively, with a transition to oral antibiotics upon discharge. Common regimens include ceftriaxone plus metronidazole or amoxicillin-clavulanate, typically for 5–7 days.

2.9.3.3 Wound care and activity restrictions

Patients are instructed to keep surgical wounds clean and dry, with special attention to laparoscopic port sites or open incisions. Showering is generally permitted within 24–48 h, but immersion in baths, swimming pools, or hot tubs should be avoided until the incisions are fully healed. Stitches or staples, if present, are typically removed in follow-up visits within 7–14 days.

Physical activity restrictions depend on the surgical technique. Light activities such as walking are encouraged early to promote circulation and prevent complications like DVT. However, strenuous exercise, heavy lifting, and abdominal straining should be avoided for at least 2–4 weeks after laparoscopic surgery and 4–6 weeks after open surgery. Patients who undergo robotic appendectomy often have a slightly shorter recovery period due to improved tissue handling and smaller incisions.

2.9.3.4 Pain management and gastrointestinal recovery

Pain is typically mild to moderate and decreases significantly within a few days. Nonopioid pain relievers such as ibuprofen and acetaminophen are preferred, while opioids may be used for short-term relief in more painful cases. Pain that worsens or is associated with fever, severe bloating, or persistent vomiting may indicate complications such as infection or bowel obstruction and requires prompt evaluation.

Bowel function should return within a few days. Patients are advised to monitor for signs of postoperative ileus such as prolonged bloating, constipation, and inability to pass gas. A high-fiber diet and adequate hydration help prevent constipation, which can be exacerbated by opioid use.

2.9.3.5 Signs of complications

Patients are educated about warning signs that require immediate medical attention. These include persistent fever above 38 °C (100.4 °F), increasing abdominal pain, redness, or purulent discharge from incisions, significant swelling at the surgical site, nausea or vomiting preventing food intake, and inability to pass stool or gas for an extended period. Symptoms such as shortness of breath or leg swelling may indicate venous thromboembolism, requiring urgent evaluation.

2.9.3.6 Follow-up and long-term recovery

A follow-up appointment is usually scheduled within 1–2 weeks after surgery to assess wound healing, review pathology results if necessary, and address any concerns. In the absence of complications, most patients fully recover within 2–4 weeks after laparoscopic or robotic surgery and 4–6 weeks after open appendectomy.

For patients who experience chronic pain, adhesion-related complications, or post-appendectomy digestive issues, further evaluation may be needed. Although appendectomy generally does not affect long-term gastrointestinal function, some individuals report mild changes in bowel habits, which typically resolve over time. Adherence to postoperative care instructions, early mobilization, proper wound management, and timely recognition of complications are key to a successful recovery.

2.10 Rare diseases of the appendix

The vermiform appendix is primarily known for its association with appendicitis, but it can also be affected by a variety of rare diseases. Although these conditions are infrequent, they can have significant clinical implications and often pose diagnostic challenges. Below, we explore some of the most uncommon diseases affecting the appendix.

2.10.1 Appendiceal diverticulosis and diverticulitis

Diverticulosis of the appendix is a relatively rare condition characterized by the formation of small outpouchings, or diverticula, in the appendiceal mucosa that protrude through the muscular layer of the appendix wall. These diverticula are thought to arise due to increased intraluminal pressure or weakness in the appendiceal wall, although the exact etiology remains unclear. In most cases, diverticulosis of the appendix is asymptomatic and is often discovered incidentally during imaging studies, surgical procedures, or pathological examination of the appendix following removal. However, when symptoms do occur, they are typically related to complications such as inflammation or infection.

One such complication is appendiceal diverticulitis, which occurs when the diverticula become inflamed or infected. This condition can present with symptoms that closely mimic those of acute appendicitis, including right lower quadrant abdominal pain, fever, nausea, and leukocytosis. However, appendiceal diverticulitis has been reported to carry a higher risk of perforation compared to classic appendicitis. This increased risk is attributed to the thinner wall of the diverticula, which is more susceptible to rupture under pressure from inflammation or infection. Perforation can lead to serious complications, such as peritonitis, abscess formation, or sepsis, making prompt diagnosis and treatment critical.

Diagnosing appendiceal diverticulitis can be challenging due to its clinical similarity to acute appendicitis. Imaging modalities such as ultrasound, CT scans, or MRI may help differentiate between the two conditions, although definitive diagnosis is often made during surgery or through histopathological examination of the removed appendix. Treatment typically involves surgical removal of the appendix (appendectomy), often performed laparoscopically, along with appropriate antibiotic therapy to address any infection.

Given the higher risk of complications associated with appendiceal diverticulitis, early recognition and intervention are essential to prevent adverse outcomes. Further research is needed to better understand the pathophysiology, risk factors, and optimal management strategies for this uncommon but potentially serious condition.

2.10.2 Endometriosis of the appendix

Endometriosis, a condition characterized by the presence of ectopic endometrial tissue outside the uterine cavity, can rarely involve the appendix. While endometriosis most commonly affects the pelvic organs, such as the ovaries, fallopian tubes, and peritoneum, it can also occur in extrapelvic sites, including the gastrointestinal tract. The appendix is one such site, though appendiceal endometriosis is uncommon, accounting for a small percentage of cases. It is most frequently observed in women of reproductive age, typically between 25 and 45 years old, reflecting the hormone-dependent nature of the disease.

The clinical presentation of appendiceal endometriosis can vary. Some patients may remain asymptomatic, with the condition being discovered incidentally during imaging, surgery, or pathological examination. However, when symptoms do occur, they often mimic other common conditions. For instance, appendiceal endometriosis can present with symptoms resembling acute appendicitis, such as right lower quadrant abdominal pain, nausea, vomiting, and fever. Alternatively, it may cause chronic right lower quadrant pain, which can be intermittent or persistent. In some cases, the pain may exhibit a cyclic pattern, worsening during menstruation due to hormonal fluctuations that cause the ectopic endometrial tissue to bleed and inflame. This cyclic pain can help differentiate endometriosis from other causes of abdominal pain, though it is not always present.

Diagnosing appendiceal endometriosis preoperatively is challenging due to its nonspecific symptoms and rarity. Imaging studies, such as ultrasound, CT, or MRI, may show abnormalities in the appendix, but these findings are often nonspecific and can be mistaken for other conditions, such as appendicitis or appendiceal tumors. As a result, the diagnosis is frequently made postoperatively, following an appendectomy or other surgical procedure, through histopathological examination of the removed tissue. Microscopic analysis typically reveals the presence of endometrial glands and stroma within the appendiceal wall, confirming the diagnosis.

Treatment for appendiceal endometriosis depends on the severity of symptoms and the extent of disease. In symptomatic cases, surgical removal of the appendix (appendectomy) is often performed, particularly if there is concern for acute appendicitis or other complications. In cases where endometriosis is more widespread, additional surgical intervention or hormonal therapy may be necessary to manage the disease. Hormonal treatments, such as oral contraceptives, gonadotropin-releasing hormone agonists, or progestins, can help suppress the growth of ectopic endometrial tissue and alleviate symptoms.

Although appendiceal endometriosis is rare, it is an important consideration in the differential diagnosis of right lower quadrant pain in women of reproductive age, particularly those with a history of endometriosis. Increased awareness of this condition can aid in timely diagnosis and appropriate management, improving patient outcomes. Further research is needed to better understand the pathogenesis, risk factors, and optimal treatment strategies for appendiceal endometriosis.

2.10.3 Amyloidosis of the appendix

Amyloidosis is a group of disorders characterized by the abnormal extracellular deposition of amyloid proteins, which are misfolded proteins that form insoluble fibrils, in various tissues and organs throughout the body. While amyloidosis can affect virtually any organ, involvement of the appendix is rare and typically occurs in the context of systemic amyloidosis, where multiple organs are affected. Localized amyloidosis of the appendix is even less common. The condition can be asymptomatic and discovered incidentally during imaging, surgery, or pathological examination, or it may present with symptoms that mimic other appendiceal pathologies, such as acute appendicitis.

The clinical presentation of appendiceal amyloidosis varies depending on the extent and location of amyloid deposition. In some cases, patients may remain entirely asymptomatic, with the condition being identified only after an appendectomy performed for unrelated reasons. However, when symptoms do occur, they often resemble those of acute appendicitis including right lower quadrant abdominal pain, nausea, vomiting, and fever. This overlap in symptoms can make preoperative diagnosis challenging, as imaging studies may not reliably distinguish amyloidosis from other causes of appendiceal inflammation or obstruction.

Definitive diagnosis of appendiceal amyloidosis relies on histological analysis. Tissue samples obtained during surgery or biopsy are stained with Congo red, a dye that binds specifically to amyloid fibrils, producing an apple-green birefringence under polarized light microscopy. This staining pattern is pathognomonic for amyloidosis and confirms the diagnosis. Further characterization of the amyloid type (e.g., AL amyloidosis, AA amyloidosis, or others) may require additional immunohistochemical or biochemical techniques, as the underlying cause of amyloid deposition can vary. AL amyloidosis, for example, is associated with plasma cell dyscrasias and the deposition of immunoglobulin light chains, while AA amyloidosis is linked to chronic inflammatory conditions and involves serum amyloid A protein.

The management of appendiceal amyloidosis depends on whether it is localized or part of systemic disease. In cases of localized amyloidosis confined to the appendix, surgical removal of the appendix (appendectomy) is typically curative and sufficient. However, if amyloidosis is systemic, treatment focuses on addressing the underlying cause and managing organ involvement. For example, in AL amyloidosis, chemotherapy or targeted therapies may be used to suppress the production of abnormal immunoglobulin light chains, while in AA amyloidosis, controlling the underlying inflammatory condition is paramount.

Although appendiceal amyloidosis is rare, it is an important consideration in the differential diagnosis of appendiceal pathology, particularly in patients with known systemic amyloidosis or those presenting with atypical symptoms. Early diagnosis and appropriate management are crucial to prevent complications and improve outcomes. Further research is needed to better understand the pathogenesis, risk factors, and optimal treatment strategies for this uncommon condition.

2.10.4 Appendiceal mucocele

Appendiceal mucocele is a rare condition characterized by the abnormal accumulation of mucus within the appendix, typically caused by obstruction due to neoplastic or non-neoplastic processes. Non-neoplastic causes include mucosal hyperplasia or obstruction from fecaliths or strictures, while neoplastic causes range from benign mucinous cystadenomas to malignant mucinous cystadenocarcinomas or low-grade appendiceal mucinous neoplasms. Symptoms, when present, may include right lower quadrant pain, a palpable mass, or nonspecific gastrointestinal complaints, though many cases are asymptomatic and discovered incidentally. A serious complication is rupture, which can lead to pseudomyxoma peritonei, a condition where mucinous material spreads throughout the peritoneal cavity, often requiring aggressive surgical and chemotherapeutic interventions. Diagnosis relies on imaging studies like ultrasound, CT, or MRI, with confirmation through histopathological examination. Treatment typically involves surgical resection, with the extent of surgery depending on the underlying cause and the presence of complications. Prognosis varies, with benign cases having excellent outcomes, while malignant or complicated cases require careful management and long-term follow-up.

2.10.5 Tuberculosis of the appendix

Tuberculosis (TB) can involve the appendix, although this is a rare manifestation of the disease and typically occurs as part of abdominal TB or disseminated TB. Abdominal TB itself is a form of extrapulmonary TB that can affect various organs within the abdomen, including the intestines, peritoneum, lymph nodes, and, less commonly, the appendix. Appendiceal TB is often secondary to the spread of *Mycobacterium tuberculosis* from a primary focus, such as the lungs or gastrointestinal tract, via hematogenous, lymphatic, or direct extension. Patients with appendiceal TB may present with a variety of symptoms, which can make diagnosis challenging. These symptoms often mimic those of acute appendicitis, including right lower quadrant abdominal pain, fever, nausea, vomiting, and leukocytosis. In other cases, patients may experience chronic abdominal pain, which can be intermittent or persistent, or present with an abdominal mass due to inflammation, abscess formation, or lymphadenopathy. The clinical presentation can overlap with other conditions, such as Crohn's disease, malignancy, or other infectious processes, necessitating a high index of suspicion, particularly in regions where TB is endemic or in patients with risk factors such as immunosuppression, previous TB exposure, or a history of living in or traveling to high-prevalence areas.

Diagnosis of appendiceal TB relies on a combination of clinical, radiological, and histopathological findings. Imaging studies, such as ultrasound or CT scans, may reveal thickening of the appendiceal wall, lymphadenopathy, or abscess formation, but these findings are nonspecific and can be seen in other conditions. Definitive diagnosis is typically made through histopathological examination of tissue samples obtained during surgery or biopsy. Histopathology often reveals characteristic caseating granulomas, which are a hallmark of TB, consisting of central necrotic material surrounded by epithelioid macrophages, lymphocytes, and multinucleated giant cells. To confirm the presence of *Mycobacterium tuberculosis*, special staining techniques such as acid-fast bacilli staining are used, which can identify the bacteria under microscopy. Additionally, molecular diagnostic methods, such as PCR testing, can detect mycobacterial DNA with high sensitivity and specificity, providing a more rapid and accurate diagnosis compared to traditional culture methods, which can take several weeks.

Treatment of appendiceal TB involves a combination of surgical and medical management. In cases where the diagnosis is made preoperatively and there is no evidence of complications such as perforation or abscess formation, antitubercular therapy (ATT) may be initiated without surgery. However, in many cases, the diagnosis is made postoperatively following an appendectomy performed for suspected acute appendicitis. Once the diagnosis is confirmed, patients should be started on a standard multidrug ATT regimen, typically consisting of isoniazid, rifampin, pyrazinamide, and ethambutol for an initial intensive phase, followed by a continuation phase with isoniazid and rifampin. The total duration of treatment is usually 6–9 months, depending on the extent of disease and the patient's response to therapy. Surgical intervention may also be required to manage complications such as abscesses, fistulas, or bowel obstruction.

The prognosis for appendiceal TB is generally favorable with timely diagnosis and appropriate treatment. However, delays in diagnosis or inadequate treatment can lead to complications such as perforation, peritonitis, or the development of fistulas, which can increase morbidity and mortality. Additionally, patients with underlying immunosuppression, such as those with HIV infection, may have a more complicated clinical course and require closer monitoring. Increased awareness of this rare presentation of TB, particularly in endemic regions or high-risk populations, is essential for early recognition and management. Further research is needed to better understand the epidemiology, clinical features, and optimal treatment strategies for appendiceal TB as well as to improve diagnostic methods to facilitate earlier and more accurate diagnosis.

2.10.6 Actinomycosis of the appendix

Actinomycosis is a rare, chronic bacterial infection caused by *Actinomyces* species, most commonly *Actinomyces israelii*, which are gram-positive, anaerobic, filamentous bacteria that normally reside in the oral cavity, gastrointestinal tract, and female genital tract. When these bacteria invade tissues, typically following mucosal injury or surgery, they can cause suppurative and granulomatous inflammation, leading to the formation of abscesses, sinus tracts, and fistulae. Appendiceal actinomycosis is an uncommon manifestation of this infection, often resulting from the spread of the bacteria to the appendix either through direct extension from adjacent structures or hematogenous dissemination. The condition is characterized by chronic inflammation of the appendix, which can lead to the development of abscesses, fistulae, or even a palpable abdominal mass. These features can closely mimic those of malignancy or other inflammatory conditions, such as Crohn's disease or TB, making clinical diagnosis challenging.

Patients with appendiceal actinomycosis may present with nonspecific symptoms, such as chronic right lower quadrant abdominal pain, fever, weight loss, or a palpable mass. In some cases, the infection may spread to surrounding tissues, leading to complications such as peritonitis, bowel obstruction, or the formation of fistulae between the appendix and adjacent organs, such as the bladder or intestines. Due to its indolent and insidious nature, the diagnosis is often delayed, and the condition is frequently mistaken for other diseases, including appendiceal tumors or chronic appendicitis. Imaging studies, such as ultrasound, CT, or MRI, may reveal thickening of the appendiceal wall, abscess formation, or fistulous tracts, but these findings are nonspecific and cannot confirm the diagnosis.

Definitive diagnosis of appendiceal actinomycosis requires histological examination of tissue samples obtained through surgery or biopsy. The hallmark finding is the presence of sulfur granules, which are yellowish, granular aggregates of bacterial filaments surrounded by inflammatory cells. These granules are pathognomonic for actinomycosis and are best visualized with special stains such as Gram stain or Grocott's methenamine silver stain. Additionally, microbiological culture of the tissue samples can help identify the causative *Actinomyces* species, although the slow-growing and fastidious nature of these bacteria often makes culture challenging.

Treatment of appendiceal actinomycosis involves a combination of surgical intervention and prolonged antibiotic therapy. Surgical removal of the affected appendix, along with drainage of any abscesses or fistulae, is often necessary to control the infection and prevent complications. Following surgery, patients are typically treated with high-dose penicillin or amoxicillin for an extended period, often ranging from 6 to 12 months, to ensure complete eradication of the bacteria. In cases of penicillin allergy, alternative antibiotics such as tetracyclines, erythromycin, or clindamycin may be used. The prognosis for appendiceal actinomycosis is generally favorable with timely diagnosis and appropriate treatment, although delays in diagnosis or inadequate therapy can lead to recurrent infections or chronic complications.

Given its rarity and nonspecific presentation, appendiceal actinomycosis requires a high index of suspicion, particularly in patients with a history of abdominal surgery, trauma, or chronic inflammatory conditions. Increased awareness of this condition among clinicians, along with careful histological and microbiological evaluation, is essential for accurate diagnosis and effective management. Further research is needed to better understand the epidemiology, risk factors, and optimal treatment strategies for this uncommon but clinically significant infection.

2.11 Misdiagnosis and legal implications

2.11.1 Introduction

Acute appendicitis is one of the most common surgical emergencies, yet its diagnosis remains a challenge. Despite advancements in imaging techniques and clinical scoring systems, misdiagnosis still occurs, leading to significant medical and legal consequences. Cases of misdiagnosis typically fall into two categories: false positives, where patients undergo unnecessary appendectomies, and false negatives, where a missed diagnosis results in complications such as perforation, peritonitis, or sepsis.

The consequences of misdiagnosing appendicitis extend beyond patient morbidity and mortality; they also have substantial legal implications. Malpractice claims related to appendicitis often involve allegations of delayed diagnosis, failure to recognize atypical presentations, and misinterpretation of imaging studies. In many cases, litigation hinges on whether the standard of care was met, and whether diagnostic errors were preventable.

This section explores the underlying causes of diagnostic errors and their medicolegal ramifications. By examining these cases, we can better understand the challenges clinicians face and the measures that can be taken to reduce diagnostic errors, ultimately improving patient outcomes and minimizing legal risks.

2.11.2 Causes of diagnostic errors

Diagnostic errors in acute appendicitis arise from a combination of patient-related, clinician-related, and system-related factors, each contributing in different ways to misdiagnosis. Patients may present with atypical symptoms, particularly if they are elderly, pediatric, pregnant, or immunocompromised. The anatomical position of the appendix can also lead to confusion; a retrocecal appendix may not cause the classic right lower quadrant pain, while a pelvic appendix can mimic gynecological or urinary conditions. Comorbidities further complicate the picture by masking inflammatory responses, and delays in seeking medical attention allow the disease to progress, sometimes making it more difficult to distinguish appendicitis from its complications or from other abdominal pathologies.

Clinician-related factors play a significant role in diagnostic errors. Many doctors rely too heavily on classical symptoms, assuming that all patients will present with periumbilical pain migrating to the right lower quadrant, associated with nausea and rebound tenderness. However, some cases may not follow this pattern, leading to missed diagnoses. Laboratory findings, while useful, can be misleading, as leukocytosis and elevated inflammatory markers are not always present in early appendicitis, nor are they specific. Inadequate physical examination can also contribute to errors, as failing to assess for Rovsing's sign, psoas sign, or obturator sign may result in overlooking a case that does not present with obvious tenderness. Cognitive biases further complicate decision-making. Anchoring bias leads clinicians to fixate on an initial incorrect diagnosis, such as gastroenteritis, even when new evidence suggests otherwise. Availability bias causes doctors to be influenced by recent experiences, diagnosing what they have seen frequently, rather than considering the full spectrum of possibilities. Premature closure, another common error, results in a failure to explore alternative diagnoses once an initial impression has been formed.

Systemic issues within healthcare settings exacerbate the problem. In many hospitals, access to imaging is limited, causing delays in obtaining ultrasound or CT scans that could confirm or rule out appendicitis. Emergency department overcrowding places pressure on clinicians to make rapid decisions, increasing the likelihood of errors. The absence of standardized diagnostic protocols leads to variability in practice, meaning that the same patient might receive different evaluations depending on the hospital or physician. Communication failures between providers further contribute to misdiagnosis, particularly during patient handoffs or when radiology reports are misinterpreted.

Even when imaging is available, it is not infallible. Ultrasound, while a useful first-line tool, is highly operator-dependent, with accuracy varying based on the experience of the person performing the scan. CT scans are more reliable, but overreliance on imaging can lead to missed cases when clinical suspicion is high but imaging appears normal. Subtle early-stage appendicitis might not be evident on a scan, and an inexperienced radiologist may misinterpret findings either overcalling or undercalling the diagnosis.

Further complicating the picture is the presence of numerous conditions that can mimic appendicitis. Gastrointestinal disorders such as gastroenteritis, Crohn's disease, diverticulitis, and Meckel's diverticulitis can present with overlapping symptoms. Gynecological conditions, including ovarian torsion, ruptured ovarian cysts, ectopic pregnancy, and PID, frequently lead to diagnostic confusion, particularly in reproductive-age women. Urological conditions like ureterolithiasis or pyelonephritis may also be mistaken for appendicitis, while inflammatory and infectious diseases such as mesenteric adenitis or tuberculous ileitis can further obscure the diagnosis.

Addressing these diagnostic challenges requires a multifaceted approach. Clinical scoring systems, such as the Alvarado score and the AIR score, provide structured decision-making tools that help reduce reliance on subjective judgment. Improved imaging protocols, including the use of contrast-enhanced CT or expert-performed ultrasound, can enhance diagnostic accuracy, particularly in ambiguous cases. Standardized diagnostic pathways help create consistency in clinical practice, ensuring that patients receive uniform evaluation regardless of the setting. Additionally, ongoing training and education for clinicians are crucial, emphasizing awareness of atypical presentations and the cognitive biases that lead to errors. By integrating these strategies, the likelihood of misdiagnosing acute appendicitis can be significantly reduced, improving patient outcomes and reducing unnecessary surgeries or delays in treatment.

2.11.3 Medicolegal aspects

The medicolegal implications of misdiagnosing appendicitis can be significant, as errors in diagnosis may lead to serious patient harm, malpractice claims, and legal consequences for healthcare providers. Appendicitis is a common surgical emergency, and delays or errors in its diagnosis can result in complications such as perforation, peritonitis, sepsis, and even death. From a legal standpoint, the failure to diagnose appendicitis in a timely manner is one of the most frequent causes of litigation in emergency medicine and general surgery. One of the primary legal concerns arises from delayed diagnosis. If a clinician fails to recognize appendicitis early and the disease progresses to perforation, leading to prolonged hospitalization, sepsis, or additional surgeries, the patient may have grounds for a malpractice lawsuit. Courts often assess whether the standard of care was breached, meaning whether a reasonably competent physician in a similar situation would have made the correct diagnosis. If it is determined that the physician deviated from accepted medical practice – such as failing to order appropriate imaging, dismissing a patient's complaints without thorough evaluation, or misinterpreting test results – they may be held legally accountable. Conversely, overdiagnosis and unnecessary surgery can also lead to legal repercussions. If a patient undergoes an appendectomy based on an incorrect diagnosis and later experiences complications such as SSIs, bowel obstruction, or anesthesia-related issues, they may claim that the procedure was unwarranted and caused avoidable harm. Negative appendectomy rates, particularly in women and children, have been a source of medicolegal scrutiny, as unnecessary surgery can expose patients to risks without any benefit. Another important issue is informed consent and communication. If a clinician fails to properly explain the risks of misdiagnosis, does not adequately discuss the possibility of appendicitis when discharging a patient with non-specific abdominal pain, or does not provide clear follow-up instructions, legal liability may arise. Patients who are sent home without appropriate warnings may deteriorate and return in critical condition, leading to allegations of negligence. Systemic factors also contribute to medicolegal risks. Emergency department overcrowding, reliance on inexperienced providers, and miscommunication between physicians, radiologists, and surgeons can lead to errors that become the basis for litigation. Hospitals may face institutional liability if systemic failures – such as lack of access to timely imaging or inadequate triage procedures – are found to contribute to a misdiagnosis. To mitigate medicolegal risks, physicians should adhere to evidence-based guidelines, document clinical reasoning thoroughly, ensure proper use of diagnostic tools, and maintain clear communication with patients. When there is uncertainty in diagnosis, arranging close follow-up or obtaining second opinions can help reduce the risk of adverse outcomes and legal claims.

2.11.4 Ethical considerations

Ethical considerations in urgent surgeries like appendectomy revolve around principles of beneficence, nonmaleficence, patient autonomy, and justice. Physicians must act swiftly to provide life-saving intervention while ensuring that decisions are based on the best available evidence and patient welfare. Informed consent remains a fundamental ethical obligation, yet in emergency situations, patients may be unable to fully comprehend or provide consent due to pain, distress, or altered mental status. When immediate surgery is necessary to prevent life-threatening complications, physicians may proceed under implied consent, prioritizing the patient's best interest. However, efforts should always be made to involve the patient or their surrogates in decision-making whenever possible. Ethical dilemmas may arise in cases of diagnostic uncertainty, where unnecessary surgery carries risks, yet delaying intervention could lead to perforation and sepsis. In resource-limited settings, ethical concerns about the fair allocation of operating room availability and surgical expertise also come into play. Additionally, vulnerable populations, such as children, the elderly, or those with cognitive impairments, require special ethical considerations to ensure their rights and well-being are safeguarded. Upholding transparency, thorough documentation, and open communication with patients and families helps navigate these ethical challenges while maintaining trust in medical decision-making.

References

–   Masson, M.P. Les lésions nerveuses de l'appendicite chronique. 262–264.
–   Carras R, F.M. A clinical and radiographic study of appendiceal fecaliths: A review of the literature and report of seven cases. Ann Surg. 1960; 151: 374–78.
–   Baron E, B.R. T, J. A microbiological comparison between acute and complicated appendicitis. Clin Infect Dis. 1992; 14: 227–31.
–   Sammalkorpi HE, M.P. L, A. A new adult appendicitis score improves diagnostic accuracy of acute appendicitis: A prospective study. BMC Gastroenterology. 2014; 14: 114.
–   A A. A practical score for the early diagnosis of acute appendicitis. Ann Emerg Med. 1986; 15: 557–64.
–   Paajanen H, G.n.J. R, T. A prospective randomized controlled multicenter trial comparing antibiotic therapy with appendectomy in the treatment of uncomplicated acute appendicitis (APPAC trial. BMC Surg. 2013; 13: 3.
–   B AC, C.I. GA. Abdominal drainage after laparoscopic appendectomy in children: An endless controversy?. Scand J Surg. 2018; 107: 197–200.

– G. GV. Acute amebic appendicitis. World J Surg. 2006; 30: 1038–42.
– MD S. Acute appendicitis. J Paediatr Child Health. 2017; 53: 1071–76.
– Eryilmaz R, S.M. B, G A, O K, B. Acute appendicitis during pregnancy. Dig Surg. 2002; 19: 40–44.
– Kong VY, B.B. ANL. Acute appendicitis in a developing country. World J Surg. 2012; 36: 2068–73.
– Caruso AM, P.A. G, R A, P P, M C, A M, et al. Acute appendicitis in children: Not only surgical treatment. J Pediatr Surg. 2017; 52: 444–48.
– Kong VY, S.B. C, D.L. Acute appendicitis in the developing world is a morbid disease. Ann R Coll Surg Engl. 2015; 97: 390–95.
– Tind S, Q.N. Acute appendicitis: A weak concordance between perioperative diagnosis, pathology and peritoneal fluid cultivation. World J Surg. 2017; 41: 70–74.
– Wray CJ, K.L. M, S.G. Acute appendicitis: Controversies in diagnosis and management. Curr Probl Surg. 2013; 50: 54–86.
– Morino M, P.L. C, E F, E M, P. Acute nonspecific abdominal pain: A randomized, controlled trial comparing early laparoscopy versus clinical observation. Ann Surg. 2006; 244: 881–86.
– Apisarnthanarak P, S.V. P, P. Alvarado score: Can it reduce unnecessary CT scans for evaluation of acute appendicitis? Am J Emerg Med. 2015; 33: 266–70.
– Otan E, A.S. K, C. Amebic acute appendicitis: Systematic review of 174 cases. World J Surg. 2013; 37: 2061–73.
– Vons C, B.C. M, S. Amoxicillin plus clavulanic acid versus appendicectomy for treatment of acute uncomplicated appendicitis: An open-label, non-inferiority, randomised controlled trial. Lancet. 2011; 377: 1573–79.
– Bulian DR, K.G. M, R. Analysis of the first 217 appendectomies of the German NOTES registry. Ann Surg. 2017; 265: 534–38.
– A S. Anemia in the critically ill. Crit Care Clin. 2004; 20: 159–78.
– Salminen P, P.H. R, T. Antibiotic therapy vs appendectomy for treatment of uncomplicated acute appendicitis: The APPAC randomized clinical trial. JAMA. 2015; 313: 2340–48.
– Andersen BR, K.F. A, H.K. Antibiotics versus placebo for prevention of postoperative infection after appendicectomy. Cochrane Database Syst Rev. 2005; 3: 001439.
– Humes D, S.W. S, J. Appendicitis. BMJ Clin Evid. 2007; 357–408.
– Ali N, A.S. Appendicitis and its surgical management experience at the University of Maiduguri Teaching Hospital Nigeria. Niger J Med. 2012; 21: 223–26.
– Brown JJ, W.C. C, S. Appendicitis in pregnancy: An ongoing diagnostic dilemma. Colorectal Dis. 2009; 11: 116–22.
– Fraser N, G.C. S, M.D. Appendicular colic and the noninflamed appendix: Fact or fiction?. Eur J Pediatr Surg. 2004; 14: 21–24.
– Ahmed K, C.T. B, K. Are wound ring protectors effective in reducing surgical site infection post appendectomy? A systematic review and meta-analysis. Ir J Med Sci. 2016; 185: 35–42.
– Barroso TVV, S.P. P, A. Assessment of the vasoactive intestinal polypeptide in morphologically normal appendices removed from patients with clinical diagnosis of acute appendicitis. Emerg Med. 2015; 5: 1–4.
– Rogozov V, B.N. Auto-appendectomy in the Antarctic: Case report. BMJ. 2009; 3394965.
– Thadepalli H, M.A. C, S.K. Bacteriology of the appendix and the ileum in health and in appendicitis. Am Surg. 1991; 57: 317–22.
– Forbes GB, L.-D.R. Calculous disease of the vermiform appendix. Gut. 1966; 7: 583–892.
– R U. Cholestasis effects of Escherichia coli endotoxin on the isolated perfused rat liver. Gatroenterology. 1976; 70: 248–53.
– Kubota Y, P.R. O, CA T, RR F, RG F, C. Colonic vasoactive intestinal peptide nerves in inflammatory bowel disease. Gastroenterology. 1992; 102: 1242–51.

– Reddy S, Tote D, Zade A, Sudabattula K, Dahmiwal T, Hatewar A, et al. Comparative analysis of robotic-assisted versus laparoscopic appendectomy: A review. Cureus. 2024 Jun; 16(6): e63488.

– Ingraham AM, C.M. B, K.Y. Comparison of outcomes after laparoscopic versus open appendectomy for acute appendicitis at 222 ACS NSQIP hospitals. Surgery. 2010; 148: 625–35.

– W S. Cope's Early Diagnosis of the Acute Abdomen. ed, editor. New York: Oxford University Press, 2010.

– Jackson HT, M.E. D, K.P. Culture-independent evaluation of the appendix and rectum microbiomes in children with and without appendicitis. PLoS One. 2014; 9: 95414.

– Prystowsky JB, P.C. N, A.P. Current problems in surgery. Appendicitis Curr Probl Surg. 2005; 42: 688–742.

– Thomas SE, D.D. C, M.H. Delayed pathology of the appendiceal stump: A case report of stump appendicitis and review. Am Surg. 1994; 60: 842–44.

– Chong CF, A.M. T, A. Development of the RIPASA score: A new appendicitis scoring system for the diagnosis of acute appendicitis. Singapore Med J. 2010; 51: 220–25.

– Solomkin JS, M.J. B, J.S. Diagnosis and management of complicated intra-abdominal infection in adults and children: guidelines by the surgical infection society and the infectious diseases society of America. Clin Infect Dis. 2010; 50: 133–64.

– Seo H, L.K. K, HJ K, K K, S-B K, S.Y. Diagnosis of acute appendicitis with sliding slab ray-sum interpretation of low-dose unenhanced CT and standard-dose IV contrast-enhanced CT scans. AJR Am J Roentgenol. 2009; 193: 96–105.

– Ruber M, B.A. E, C O, G A, R.E. Different cytokine profiles in patients with a history of gangrenous or phlegmonous appendicitis. Clin Exp Immunol. 2006; 143: 117–24.

– Bliss D, M.J. CD. Discordance of the pediatric surgeon's intraoperative assessment of pediatric appendicitis with the pathologists report. J Pediatr Surg. 2010; 45: 1398–403.

– **Ranji** GL, Simel DL, Shojania KG. Do opiates affect the clinical evaluation of patients with acute abdominal pain?. JAMA. 2006; 296(14): 1764–74.

– Kulik DM, U.E. M, J.L. Does this child have appendicitis? A systematic review of clinical prediction rules for children with acute abdominal pain. J Clin Epidemiol. 2013; 66: 95–104.

– Raval MV, L.T. R, M. Dollars and sense of interval appendectomy in children: A cost analysis. J Pediatr Surg. 2010; 45: 1817–25.

– Sippola S, G.J. T, R. Economic evaluation of antibiotic therapy versus appendicectomy for the treatment of uncomplicated acute appendicitis from the APPAC randomized clinical trial. Br J Surg. 2017; 104: 1355–61.

– Kim M, K.S. C, H.J. Effect of surgical timing and outcomes for appendicitis severity. Ann Surg Treat Res. 2016; 357: 357–85.

– Georgiou R, E.S. S, MP P, A H, N.J. Efficacy and safety of nonoperative treatment for acute appendicitis: A meta-analysis. Pediatrics. 2017; 139: 20163003.

– Artifon ELA, U.R. FJ, C.K. Endoluminal appendectomy: The first description in humans for acute appendicitis. Endoscopy. 2017; 49: 609–10.

– K. S. Endoscopic appendectomy. Endoscopy. 1983; 357: 59–64.

– Trejo-Ávila ME, R.-L.S. CL, E. Enhanced recovery after surgery protocol allows ambulatory laparoscopic appendectomy in uncomplicated acute appendicitis: A prospective, randomized trial. Surg Endosc. 2019; 33: 429–36.

– Livingston EH, F.T. W, WA H, R.W. Epidemiological similarities between appendicitis and diverticulitis suggesting a common underlying pathogenesis. Arch Surg. 2011; 146: 308–14.

– Platon A, J.H. R, O B, C V, F G, P. Evaluation of a low-dose CT protocol with oral contrast for assessment of acute appendicitis. Eur Radiol. 2009; 19: 446–54.

– Collaborative. Rsg. Evaluation of appendicitis risk prediction models in adults with suspected appendicitis: Identifying adults at low risk of appendicitis. Br J Surg. 2019.

–   Salo M, M.N. R, B. Evaluation of the microbiome in children's appendicitis. Int J Colorectal Dis. 2017; 32: 19–28.
–   Nemeth L, O 'Briain DS, M, M P,P. Evidence of an inflammatory pathologic condition in "normal" appendices following emergency appendectomy. Arch Pathol Lab Med. 2001; 125: 759–64.
–   Anderson JE, B.S. C, D.C. Examining a common disease with unknown etiology: Trends in epidemiology and surgical management of appendicitis in California, 1995–2009. World J Surg. 2012; 36: 2787–94.
–   Bouchard S, R.P. R, AP A, N.S. Expression of neuropeptides in normal and abnormal appendices. J Pediatr Surg. 2001; 36: 1222–26.
–   O SA, A.-S.A. LH. Genetic and environmental influences on the risk of acute appendicitis in twins. Br J Surg. 2009; 357: 1336–40.
–   Silva FR, d.R.M. S, B.R. Hyperbilirubinaemia alone cannot distinguish a perforation in acute appendicitis. ANZ J Surg. 2016; 86: 255–59.
–   Chaudhary P, **A.K. NS,** Biswal UC. Hyperbilirubinemia as a predictor of gangrenous/perforated appendicitis: A prospective study. Ann Gastroenterol. 2013; 26: 325–31.
–   MA B. Imaging acute appendicitis. Semin Ultrasound CT MR. 2008; 29: 293–307.
–   Khandelwal A, F.N. K, A. Imaging of acute abdomen in pregnancy. Radiol Clin North Am. 2013; 24: 1005–22.
–   Busch M, G.F. A, S K, R M, U Z, U. In-hospital delay increases the risk of perforation in adults with appendicitis. World J Surg. 2011; 357: 1626–33.
–   Wang HT, S.H. Incidental appendectomy in the era of managed care and laparoscopy. J Am Coll Surg. 2001; 192: 182–88.
–   Andersson R, H.A. T, A N, PO O, G. Indications for operation in suspected appendicitis and incidence of perforation. BMJ. 1994; 308: 107–10.
–   Wallace CA, P.M. S, DI F, SJ A, SW T, A. Influence of imaging on the negative appendectomy rate in pregnancy. Gastrointest Surg. 2008; 12: 46–50.
–   Lai HW, L.C. C, J.H. Interval appendectomy after conservative treatment of an appendiceal mass. World J Surg. 2006; 30: 352–57.
–   Iqbal CW, K.E. M, V.E. Interval appendectomy after perforated appendicitis: What are the operative risks and luminal patency rates?. J Surg Res. 2012; 177: 127–30.
–   Senekjian L, N.R. B, B N, R. Interval appendectomy: Fi nding the breaking point for cost-effectiveness. J Am Coll Surg. 2016; 223: 632–43.
–   Oldmeadow C, W.I. M, K. Investigation of the relationship between smoking and appendicitis in Australian twins. Ann Epidemiol. 2008; 18: 631–36.
–   Hajibandeh S, H.S. K, A. Irrigation versus suction alone in laparoscopic appendectomy: Is dilution the solution to pollution? A systematic review and meta-analysis. Surg Innov. 2018; 25: 174–82.
–   Perrin J, M.P. U, V. Is hook diathermy safe to dissect the mesoappendix in paediatric patients? A 10-year experience. N Z Med J. 2019; 132: 41–47.
–   Myla K, Bou-Ayash N, Kim WC, Bugaev N, Bawazeer M. Is implementation of robotic-assisted procedures in acute care general surgery cost-effective?. J Robot Surg. 2024 May 27; 18(1): 223.
–   Hall NJ, J.C. E, S. Is interval appendicectomy justified after successful nonoperative treatment of an appendix mass in children? A systematic review. J Pediatr Surg. 2011; 46: 767–71.
–   Wright GP, M.M. C, J.T. Is there truly an oncologic indication for interval appendectomy?. Am J Surg. 2015; 209: 442–46.
–   Walsh CA, T.T. W SR. Laparoscopic versus open appendicectomy in pregnancy: A systematic review. Int J Surg. 2008; 6: 339–44.
–   Moore MM, K.A. H, C.S. Magnetic resonance imaging n pediatric appendicitis: A systematic review. Pediatr Radiol. 2016; 46: 928–39.

– Rushing A, B.N. J, C C, JJ F, N C, M R, et al. Management of acute appendicitis in adults: A practice management guideline from the eastern association for the surgery of Trauma. J Trauma Acute Care Surg. 2019; 87: 214–24.

– Mason RJ, M.A. S, H. Meta-analysis of randomized trials comparing antibiotic therapy with appendectomy for acute uncomplicated (no abscess or phlegmon) appendicitis. Surg Infect (Larchmt. 2012; 13: 74–84.

– RE A. Meta-analysis of the clinical and laboratory diagnosis of appendicitis. Br J Surg. 2004; 91: 28–37.

– Guinane CM, T.A. F, F. Microbial composition of human appendices from patients following appendectomy. MBio. 2013; 4: 00366–12.

– García-Marín A, P.-L.M. MG, E RC, L CR, A. Microbiologic analysis of complicated and uncomplicated acute appendicitis. Surg Infect (Larchmt. 2018; 19: 83–86.

– Dewhurst C, B.P. P, I. MRI evaluation of acute appendicitis in pregnancy. J Magn Reson Imaging. 2013; 37: 566–75.

– Collaborative. NSR. Multicentre observational study of performance variation in provision and outcome of emergency appendicectomy. Br J Surg. 2013; 1240: 1240–52.

– Wen SW, **Naylor** CD. Pitfalls in nonrandomized outcomes studies. The case of incidental appendectomy with open cholecystectomy. JAMA. 1995; 274: 1687–91.

– McGory ML, Z.D. T, A. Negative appendectomy in pregnant women is associated with a substantial risk of fetal loss. J Am Coll Surg. 2007; 205: 534–40.

– H H. Neurogene appendicopathie. Langenbecks Arch Chir. 1980; 351: 171–78.

– Olsen BS, H.S. Neurogenous hyperplasia leading to appendiceal obliteration. Histopathology. 1987; 11: 843–49.

– P S, F.T. di MFF, E W, P I, H F, MW B. Neuroimmune appendicitis. Lancet. 1999; 354: 461–66.

– Xiong S, **P.P. N**, O'Briain DS, R, D.J. Neuronal hypertrophy in acute appendicitis. Arch Pathol Lab Med. 2000; 124: 1429–33.

– Hajibandeh S, H.S. H, N M, M. Neutrophil-to-lymphocyte ratio predicts acute appendicitis and distinguishes between complicated and uncomplicated appendicitis: A systematic review and meta-analysis. Am J Surg. 2020; 219: 154–63.

– Navarra G, P.E. O, S. One-wound laparoscopic cholecystectomy. Br J Surg. 1997; 84: 695.

– Quilici PJ, Wolberg H, McConnell N. Operating costs, fiscal impact, value analysis and guidance for the routine use of robotic technology in abdominal surgical procedures. Surg Endosc. 2022 Feb; 36(2): 1433–43.

– Helling TS, S.D. S, S. Operative versus non-operative management in the care of patients with complicated appendicitis. Am J Surg. 2017; 214: 1195–200.

– Frazee RC, A.S. I, C.L. Outpatient laparoscopic appendectomy: Is it time to end the discussion?. J Am Coll Surg. 2016; 222: 473–77.

– M. S. Pediatric appendicitis score. J Pediatr Surg. 2002; 37: 877–81.

– Puri P, M.A.A.I.S.M. O, KT M, P.D.E. Pediatric Surgery and Urology: Long Term Outcomes. 2nd edn, Cambridge University Press, 2006; pp.374–84.

– Kollar D, M.D. B, M. Predicting acute appendicitis? A comparison of the Alvarado score, the Appendicitis Inflammatory Response Score and clinical assessment. World J Surg. 2015; 39: 104–09.

– Allemann P, P.H. D, N. Prevention of infectious complications after laparoscopic appendectomy for complicated acute appendicitis – The role of routine abdominal drainage. Langenbecks Arch Surg. 2011; 396: 63–68.

– Pogorelic Z, R.S. M, I J, I. Prospective validation of Alvarado score and pediatric appendicitis score for the diagnosing of acute appendicitis in children. Pediatric Emergency Care. 2015; 31: 164–68.

– Kong VY, V.d.L.S. AC. Quantifying the disparity in outcome between urban and rural patients with acute appendicitis in South Africa. S Afr Med J. 2013; 103: 742–45.

– Park HC, K.M. L, B.H. Randomized clinical trial of antibiotic therapy for uncomplicated appendicitis: Antibiotic therapy for uncomplicated appendicitis. Br J Surg. 2017; 104: 1785–90.
– Rivera-Chavez FA, W.H. LG. Regional and systemic cytokine responses to acute inflammation of the vermiform appendix. Ann Surg. 2003; 237: 408–16.
– Sanderfer VC, Jensen S, Qadri HI, Yang H, Benham EC, Lauer C, et al. Rise of the robots: Implementing robotic surgery into the acute care surgery practice. Surg Endosc. 2025 Jan; 39(1): 472–79.
– Zingone F, S.A. H, DJ W, J. Risk of acute appendicitis in and around pregnancy: A population-based cohort study from England. Ann Surg. 2015; 261: 332–37.
– KhanMS C, **N S, M T,** Memon WA, AAR. Risk of appendicitis in patients with incidentally discovered appendicoliths. J Surg Res. 2018; 221: 84–87.
– Singh JP, M.J. Role of the faecolith in modern-day appendicitis. Ann R Coll Surg Engl. 2013; 95: 48–51.
– Puapong D, L.S. H, P.I. Routine interval appendectomy in children is not indicated. J Pediatr Surg. 2007; 42: 1500–03.
– Varadhan KK, N.K. L, D.N. Safety and efficacy of antibiotics compared with appendicectomy for treatment of uncomplicated acute appendicitis: Meta-analysis of randomised controlled trials. BMJ. 2012; 344: 2156.
– Ciarrocchi A, A.G. Safety and impact on diagnostic accuracy of early analgesia in suspected acute appendicitis: A meta-analysis. Int J Surg. 2013; 11: 847–52.
– JR KJ, Fellinger E, Reed W. SAGES guideline for laparoscopic appendectomy. Surg Endosc. 2010; 24: 757–61.
– Scott A, S.S. R, J.D. Same-day discharge in laparoscopic acute non-perforated appendectomy. J Am Coll Surg. 2017; 224: 43–48.
– Chen JM, G.W. X, S.X. Single-incision versus conventional three-port laparoscopic appendectomy: A meta-analysis of randomized controlled trials. Minim Invasive Ther Allied Technol. 2015.
– Aly NE, M.D. A, EH L vs. Standard dose computed tomography in suspected acute appendicitis: Is it time for a change?. Int J Surg. 2016; 31: 71–79.
– Mangi AA, B.D. Stump appendicitis. Am Surg. 2000; 66: 739–41.
– Wilasrusmee C, S.B. M, M A, J T, A. Systematic review and meta-analysis of safety of laparoscopic versus open appendicectomy for suspected appendicitis in pregnancy. Br J Surg. 2012; 357: 1470–78.
– Ruber M, A.M. P, BF O, G A, RE E, C. Systemic Th17-like cytokine pattern in gangrenous appendicitis but not in phlegmonous appendicitis. Surgery. 2010; 147: 366–72.
– Jones RP, J.R. S, BR D, TS R, J O, E.W. The Alvarado score as a method for reducing the number of CT studies when appendiceal ultrasound fails to visualize the appendix in adults. AJR Am J Roentgenol. 2015; 204: 519–26.
– Ohle R, **O.R.F,** O 'Brien KK. The Alvarado score for predicting acute appendicitis: A systematic review. BMC Med. 2011; 9: 139.
– Andersson M, A.R. The appendicitis inflammatory response score: A tool for the diagnosis of acute appendicitis that outperforms the Alvarado score. World J Surg. 2008; 32: 1843–49.
– Mousavi SM, P.S. T, S G. The effects of intravenous acetaminophen on pain and clinical findings of patients with acute appendicitis; a randomized clinical trial. Bull Emerg Trauma. 2014; 2(1): 22–26.
– Lee JH, P.Y. C, J.S. The epidemiology of appendicitis and appendectomy in South Korea: National registry data. J Epidemiol. 2010; 20: 97–105.
– Addiss DG, S.N. F, B.S. The epidemiology of appendicitis and appendectomy in the United States. Am J Epidemiol. 1990; 132: 910–25.
– Ferris M, Q.S. K, B.S. The global incidence of appendicitis: A systematic review of population-based studies. Ann Surg. 2017; 266: 237–41.
– C. M. The indications for early laparotomy in appendicitis. Ann Surg. 1891; 357: 233–54.

– Sammalkorpi HE, M.P. S, H. The introduction of Adult Appendicitis Score reduced negative appendectomy rate. Scand J Surg. 2017; 106: 196–201.
– Obinwa O, C.M. F, J. The microbiology of bacterial peritonitis due to appendicitis in children. Irish J Med Sci. 2014; 183: 585–91.
– RE A. The natural history and traditional management of appendicitis revisited: Spontaneous resolution and predominance of prehospital perforations imply that a correct diagnosis is more important than an early diagnosis. World J Surg. 2007; 31: 86–92.
– S S, S.A. GE. The NOTA Study (Non Operative Treatment for Acute Appendicitis): Prospective study on the efficacy and safety of antibiotics (amoxicillin and clavulanic acid) for treating patients with right lower quadrant abdominal pain and long-term follow-up of conservatively treated suspected appendicitis. Ann Surg. 2014; 260: 109–17.
– Mazuski JE, T.J. M, A.K. The Surgical Infection Society revised guidelines on the management of intra-abdominal infection. Surg Infect. 2017; 18: 1–76.
– McKay R, S.J. The use of the clinical scoring system by Alvarado in the decision to perform computed tomography for acute appendicitis in the ED. Am J Emerg Med. 2007; 25: 489–93.
– Malonga EE, S.A. YJG. The value of metronidazole in the indications for appendicectomy in a tropical environment: Apropos of 183 cases. Med Trop. 1988 Mar; 48: 45–47.
– Faiz O, C.J. B, T. Traditional and laparoscopic appendectomy in adults: Outcomes in English NHS hospitals between 1996 and 2006. Ann Surg. 2008; 248: 800–8006.
– A. B. United Kingdom National Surgical Research Collaborative. Safety of short, in-hospital delays before surgery for acute appendicitis: Multicentre cohort study, systematic review, and meta-analysis. Ann Surg. 2014; 357: 894–903.
– Singal R, Z.M. S, B.P. Unusual entities of appendix mimicking appendicitis clinically. Maedica. 2017; 12: 23–29.
– Parks NA, S.T. Update on imaging for acute appendicitis. Surg Clin North Am. 2011; 91: 141–54.
– Anandalwar SP, C.M. B, R.G. Use of white blood cell count and polymorphonuclear leukocyte differential to improve the predictive value of ultrasound for suspected appendicitis in children. J Am Coll Surg. 2015; 220: 1010–17.
– Park JS, K.J. K, YJ K, W.Y. Utility of the immature granulocyte percentage for diagnosing acute appendicitis among clinically suspected appendicitis in adult. J Clin Lab Anal. 2018; 32: 22458.
– Chiarugi M, B.P. D, L. What you see is not what you get." A plea to remove a 'normal' appendix during diagnostic laparoscopy. Acta Chir Belg. 2001; 101: 243–45.
– S S, B.A. KMD. WSES Jerusalem guidelines for diagnosis and treatment of acute appendicitis. World J Emerg Surg. 2016; 11: 34.

Chapter 3
Malignancies

3.1 Primary malignancies

The first documented case of malignant disease affecting the appendix was reported by Merling in 1838, marking a significant milestone in the understanding of appendiceal pathology. Neoplasms of the appendix are particularly challenging to diagnose preoperatively, as they are rarely suspected based on clinical presentation alone. Instead, these tumors are most often identified incidentally during surgery or through postoperative pathologic examination of the removed tissue. Over time, growing awareness of appendiceal malignancies, along with advancements in understanding their pathophysiology and clinical presentation, has led to heightened interest among both surgical and medical oncologists. This increased focus has driven improvements in diagnostic techniques, treatment strategies, and patient outcomes.

The incidence of primary malignant tumors of the appendix is relatively low, estimated at approximately 0.97 cases per 100,000 individuals, based on data derived from large, nation-representative databases. Despite their rarity, these tumors are not insignificant from a clinical perspective. Neoplasia is found in about 1–2% of all appendices removed during appendectomy, a procedure that is one of the most commonly performed surgeries worldwide. Given the high frequency of appendectomies, the cumulative number of appendiceal neoplasms detected is substantial, underscoring the importance of maintaining a high index of clinical suspicion. Failure to recognize these tumors can result in missed diagnoses of potentially life-threatening conditions, emphasizing the need for thorough evaluation and histopathological examination of appendiceal specimens.

Appendiceal tumors encompass a diverse range of histological types, each with distinct characteristics and clinical implications. These include mucin-producing and non-mucin-producing adenocarcinomas, neuroendocrine tumors (NETs), goblet cell carcinomas (GCCs), lymphomas, and mesenchymal tumors. Mucin-producing adenocarcinomas are notable for their ability to secrete mucin, which can lead to pseudomyxoma peritonei (PMP), a condition characterized by the accumulation of mucinous material in the peritoneal cavity. Non-mucin-producing adenocarcinomas, on the other hand, behave more like conventional colorectal adenocarcinomas. NETs, which arise from neuroendocrine cells, are the most common type of appendiceal tumor and are often discovered incidentally during appendectomy. GCCs are rare hybrid tumors that exhibit both glandular and neuroendocrine features, presenting unique diagnostic and therapeutic challenges. Lymphomas and mesenchymal tumors of the appendix are exceedingly rare but can occur, further contributing to the complexity of appendiceal neoplasms.

https://doi.org/10.1515/9783112219782-003

The diversity of appendiceal tumors highlights the importance of accurate histopathological diagnosis and tailored treatment approaches. While some tumors, such as early-stage NETs, have an excellent prognosis, others, like advanced adenocarcinomas, can be aggressive and require multimodal therapy. The increasing recognition of these tumors, coupled with advancements in diagnostic imaging, histopathology, and treatment modalities, has improved the ability to manage these rare but clinically significant conditions effectively. As research continues to shed light on the biology and behavior of appendiceal neoplasms, the medical community is better equipped to optimize patient care and outcomes.

The incidence of mucinous tumors of the appendix in the United States has shown a notable upward trend over recent decades, accompanied by a decrease in the average age at diagnosis. This pattern suggests a shift in the epidemiology of these tumors, though the underlying reasons remain unclear. A similar trend was observed in a comprehensive registry study conducted in the Netherlands, which analyzed data from patients diagnosed between 1980 and 2010. The study revealed a comparable increase in the incidence of mucinous tumors and a younger age at diagnosis, raising questions about whether these changes reflect a true rise in the number of cases or are instead attributable to heightened clinical awareness and improved diagnostic techniques. Enhanced imaging technologies, more frequent surgical interventions, and greater pathological scrutiny may have contributed to the increased detection of these tumors, even if their actual occurrence has not significantly changed.

Appendiceal mucinous neoplasms are relatively rare, accounting for approximately 0.4% to 1% of all gastrointestinal malignancies. Despite their rarity, these tumors are clinically significant due to their potential to cause PMP, a condition characterized by the accumulation of mucin in the peritoneal cavity, which can lead to severe complications if left untreated. The age-adjusted incidence of mucinous tumors is estimated to be around 0.12 cases per 1 million individuals annually, highlighting their low prevalence in the general population.

Demographically, women represent a slight majority among those affected, comprising 50% to 55% of cases. The majority of patients diagnosed with appendiceal mucinous neoplasms are white, although no significant differences in incidence have been observed across racial or ethnic groups. Similarly, there is no notable disparity in the occurrence of these tumors between genders, suggesting that biological or environmental factors may play a more critical role in their development than sex or race.

The reasons for the observed increase in incidence and the younger age at diagnosis remain speculative. Potential explanations include changes in environmental or lifestyle factors, improved diagnostic capabilities, or even shifts in the biological behavior of the tumors themselves. Further research is needed to clarify these trends and to determine whether they reflect a true epidemiological shift or are simply the result of better detection and reporting. Understanding these patterns is crucial for guiding clinical practice, improving early diagnosis, and optimizing treatment strategies for patients with appendiceal mucinous neoplasms.

Neuroendocrine neoplasms of the appendix are a distinct group of tumors with an estimated incidence rate of 0.15 to 0.6 cases per 100,000 individuals annually. These tumors exhibit a slight female predominance in Western countries, though the reasons for this gender disparity remain unclear. While appendiceal NETs are exceptionally rare in children, they are notably one of the most common gastrointestinal neuroendocrine cancers in pediatric cohorts when they do occur. This highlights their unique epidemiological profile compared to other gastrointestinal malignancies.

The average age at diagnosis for appendiceal NETs ranges between 32 and 42 years, which contrasts sharply with epithelial tumors of the appendix. Epithelial tumors, which account for only 0.1% of epithelial malignancies in the colon and rectum, are typically diagnosed much later in life, usually beginning in the seventh decade. This difference in age distribution underscores the distinct biological behavior and origin of these two types of appendiceal tumors.

Appendiceal NETs originate from subepithelial neuroendocrine cells located in the lamina propria and submucosal layers of the appendiceal wall. These tumors are the most frequently encountered neoplasms of the appendix, identified in approximately 0.2–0.7% of all appendectomy specimens. Diagnosis is most commonly made during the second or third decade of life, often as an incidental finding during surgery for suspected appendicitis or other abdominal procedures. The majority of these tumors are detected at an early stage, which contributes to their generally favorable prognosis.

In recent years, the reported incidence of appendiceal NETs has been increasing. This trend may reflect improved diagnostic techniques, greater awareness among clinicians, and more thorough pathological examination of appendectomy specimens rather than a true rise in the number of cases. Importantly, no significant differences in incidence have been observed across racial or ethnic groups, suggesting that genetic or environmental factors specific to race do not play a major role in the development of these tumors.

Appendiceal NETs constitute the largest subgroup of primary appendiceal neoplasms, representing approximately 30–80% of all such tumors. Their incidental discovery during appendectomy or other abdominal surgeries is common in both adults and children. The prognosis for early-stage appendiceal NETs is excellent, with 5-year survival rates approaching 100%. However, when considering all tumor stages, including more advanced cases, the prognosis becomes less favorable, with 5-year survival rates ranging between 70% and 85%. This variability underscores the importance of early detection and the need for appropriate staging and management to optimize outcomes.

The increasing incidence, coupled with the generally favorable prognosis of early-stage tumors, highlights the importance of continued research and clinical vigilance. Understanding the biological behavior, risk factors, and optimal treatment strategies for appendiceal NETs is essential for improving patient care and ensuring favorable long-term outcomes.

GCC is an exceptionally rare and unique type of appendiceal cancer, accounting for approximately 14% to 19% of all primary malignancies of the appendix. This tumor is characterized by its hybrid nature, exhibiting features of both glandular epithelial and neuroendocrine differentiation, with the presence of goblet cells – specialized mucus-secreting cells typically found in the lining of the intestines. This dual composition makes GCC distinct from other appendiceal tumors and contributes to its complex clinical behavior.

Demographically, GCC is more commonly diagnosed in white individuals, with a mean age at diagnosis of 58 years. Unlike some other cancers, there is no reported difference in incidence between males and females, suggesting that gender does not play a significant role in its development. Additionally, no specific risk factors have been definitively linked to the development of goblet cell adenocarcinoma, making it challenging to identify populations at higher risk or to implement preventive measures.

Clinically, GCC often presents with symptoms that mimic acute appendicitis, such as sudden and severe abdominal pain. In fact, more than half of the cases are initially misdiagnosed as appendicitis, leading to surgical intervention during which the tumor is discovered incidentally. This overlap in presentation with a common condition like appendicitis underscores the diagnostic challenge posed by GCC and highlights the importance of thorough histopathological examination of appendectomy specimens.

The prognosis of GCC is intermediate compared to other appendiceal tumors. It is generally less aggressive than adenocarcinoma but more aggressive than NETs, which tend to follow a more indolent course. The stage at diagnosis plays a critical role in determining outcomes. Patients diagnosed with stage I or II GCC have a very good prognosis, with high survival rates following appropriate treatment. However, the prognosis deteriorates significantly for advanced-stage disease. In stage III, the 5-year overall survival drops to 22%, and in stage IV, it further declines to 14%. This stark difference in outcomes based on staging emphasizes the importance of early detection and intervention.

The management of GCC typically involves surgical resection, often accompanied by chemotherapy, particularly in advanced stages. Given its rarity and hybrid nature, treatment strategies are often tailored to the individual patient, taking into account the tumor's size, stage, and histological features. Multidisciplinary approaches involving surgeons, oncologists, and pathologists are essential to optimize care and improve outcomes.

GCC is a rare and complex appendiceal tumor with a unique histological profile and clinical behavior. While early-stage disease carries a favorable prognosis, advanced-stage GCC is associated with significantly poorer outcomes. Continued research into its biology, risk factors, and optimal treatment strategies is crucial to improving the management and survival of patients with this rare malignancy.

Primary lymphomas of the appendix are exceedingly rare, representing only 1.3% to 2.6% of all gastrointestinal lymphomas, with non-Hodgkin lymphoma (NHL) being the predominant type. These tumors typically present in younger individuals, with most cases occurring in the second and third decades of life. The reported age range for appendiceal lymphoma is broad, spanning from 4 to 70 years, with a mean age at diagnosis of 25 years. This younger age distribution distinguishes appendiceal lymphoma from other gastrointestinal malignancies, which are more commonly diagnosed in older adults. The clinical presentation often mimics acute appendicitis, leading to surgical intervention during which the diagnosis is made. Due to its rarity, the management of primary appendiceal lymphoma requires a tailored approach, often involving surgery, chemotherapy, and sometimes radiation therapy, depending on the stage and histological subtype.

Mesenchymal tumors of the appendix are also exceptionally rare, with only a limited number of case reports documented in the medical literature. Among these, gastrointestinal stromal tumors (GISTs) and leiomyomas are the most frequently reported types. GISTs, which arise from the interstitial cells of Cajal, and leiomyomas, which originate from smooth muscle cells, are the most common mesenchymal tumors affecting the appendix. However, other rare mesenchymal tumors, such as schwannomas, neurofibromas, sarcomas, and Kaposi's sarcoma, have also been described. Kaposi's sarcoma, in particular, has been reported in patients with human immunodeficiency virus (HIV) infection, reflecting the appendix's susceptibility to malignancies associated with immunosuppression. The diagnosis of these tumors is often incidental, occurring during surgery or pathological examination of the appendix, and treatment typically involves surgical resection with or without adjuvant therapy, depending on the tumor type and behavior.

In this chapter, we are going to discuss the diagnosis, clinical features, and treatment of all such malignancies.

3.1.1 Histopathology

The classification of appendiceal adenocarcinomas has been controversial and subject to several revisions. Malignancies of the appendix can be broadly classified according to their histology into epithelial and non-epithelial groups. The epithelial group encompasses adenocarcinomas, adenomas, and NETs, whereas non-epithelial tumors include lymphomas and mesenchymal tumors. Epithelial neoplasms are further subdivided based on mucin production, as there is strong evidence that it correlates with a more aggressive biologic behavior. Appendiceal mucinous neoplasms include a heterogeneous group of malignancies with highly varying malignant potentials. Mucin production can occlude the appendiceal lumen, leading to abdominal pain, with clinical features resembling acute appendicitis. Therefore, early-stage mucinous tumors are often diagnosed at appendectomy performed for suspected appendicitis. Appendiceal mucinous neoplasms are found in approximately 0.2–0.3% of specimens. Low-grade appendiceal mucinous neoplasms (LAMNs) are well-differentiated and show a slow rate of growth. They present with gradual obstruction, appendiceal dilatation, and fibrosis, leading to medical conditions previously known as mucocele or mucinous cystadenoma; such terms are now considered deprecated. In fact, they now fall under the histologic definition of low-grade appendiceal neoplasms. High-grade lesions invade the muscularis mucosa. Intraperitoneal rupture of a mucinous lesion results in peritoneal dissemination. The consequent spread on the peritoneal surface results in further production of mucin with variable cellularity, which may ultimately lead to the development of PMP. This term indicates the accumulation of mucin within the peritoneal cavity. PMP can also be secondary to other mucin-producing malignancies, such as ovarian, colonic, or pancreatic cancer. The extent of peritoneal involvement is assessed by the peritoneal carcinomatosis index (PCI), which evaluates the presence and extent of disease in each of nine abdominal areas and four small bowel segments. It is recommended to grade PMP based on the degree of cellularity within the mucin, in the following categories: acellular, low-grade histologic features, high-grade histologic features, and PMP with signet ring cells. The low-grade group roughly corresponds to the obsolete expression "disseminated peritoneal adenomucinosis", whereas peritoneal carcinomatosis is usually sustained by high-grade malignancies. However, mucinous dissemination and its various clinical expressions, such as omental caking, may represent either low- or high-grade PMP.

Nonmucinous appendiceal neoplasms share significant similarities with colorectal adenocarcinomas, both in terms of their biological behavior and treatment approaches. These tumors typically progress through three primary mechanisms: direct extension into surrounding tissues, spread via the lymphatic system, and hematogenous (blood-borne) metastases. This pattern of progression is akin to that observed in colorectal cancers, making the management strategies for nonmucinous appendiceal neoplasms closely aligned with those used for colorectal adenocarcinomas.

From a genetic standpoint, appendiceal adenocarcinomas exhibit molecular characteristics that closely resemble those of colorectal cancers. Key markers such as p53, CD44, and CDX2 are commonly expressed in both tumor types, highlighting their shared genetic pathways. The p53 protein, a well-known tumor suppressor, plays a critical role in regulating cell division and preventing cancer formation. CD44 is involved in cell adhesion and migration, while CDX2 is a transcription factor essential for intestinal development and differentiation. The presence of these markers in appendiceal adenocarcinomas underscores their genetic similarity to colorectal cancers and provides insights into their behavior and potential therapeutic targets.

Poorly differentiated nonmucinous appendiceal neoplasms, which are more aggressive in nature, often exhibit the presence of signet ring cells. These cells are characterized by their distinctive appearance, where the nucleus is pushed to the side by an accumulation of mucin, giving the cell a "signet ring" shape. Tumors containing signet ring cells are particularly aggressive, demonstrating a high propensity for local invasion and distant metastasis. This aggressive behavior often correlates with a poorer prognosis, as these tumors are more likely to spread to other organs, such as the liver, lungs, or peritoneum, complicating treatment, and reducing survival rates.

Goblet cell tumors are now considered a variant of adenocarcinoma that demonstrates features resembling both neuroendocrine cancer and adenocarcinoma, with intermediate biologic aggressiveness. For this reason, treatment is the same as for adenocarcinoma. Non-epithelial appendiceal cancers include lymphomas and mesenchymal tumors (e.g., sarcomas) that are histologically similar to their counterparts located in the rest of the gastrointestinal tract.

The diagnosis of mucinous tumors relies on the presence of mucin found on pathologic examination. Appendiceal mucinous neoplasms stain positive for CK20 and negative for CK7 in more than two-thirds of cases. Mucinous neoplasms are usually positive for MUC5AC and DPC4 as well. Notably, both colorectal and appendiceal adenocarcinoma share the same pattern of CK positivity. For this reason, it has been hypothesized that appendiceal mucinous tumors may follow the same pathogenic pathway as colorectal adenocarcinoma, which arises from adenomatous polyps with an established and predictable genetic progression in an adenoma–carcinoma sequence. These steps include the fixation of point mutations in the KRAS proto-oncogene and mutations or deletions in the TP53 gene on chromosome 17p, mutations or deletions in the adenomatous polyposis coli (APC) gene on chromosome 5q, and mutations in the beta-catenin gene. An alternative known pathway of carcinogenesis involves microsatellite instability, resulting from mutations in nucleotide mismatch repair genes, including hMSH2, hMLH1, PMS1, PMS2, and GTBP. Genetic analyses on mucin-producing adenocarcinomas of the appendix support clonality and the presence of specific molecular signatures. Observations suggest that KRAS mutations could represent an early event in the tumorigenesis of appendiceal mucinous tumors, but are insufficient per se to lead to peritoneal spread. Studies on gene expression in low-grade appendiceal cancer have identified biomarkers predictive of efficacy in patients undergoing complete debulking surgery and hyperthermic intraperitoneal chemotherapy (HIPEC), with high gene expression predicting poor survival. Genomic profiling studies of appendiceal mucinous specimens using second-generation sequencing have detected base substitutions in KRAS in a majority of cases, along with mutations in TP53, MYC, SMAD4, and APC.

In 1928, Masson first defined subepithelial cells as the origin of appendiceal NETs, proving their mixed endocrine and neural nature. The majority of neural cells are located in the tip of the appendix, whereas the epithelial neuroendocrine cells are distributed equally throughout the appendix. A clear relationship between prognosis and the exact location of the tumor in the appendix has not been established. However, neoplasms located at the base are associated with a higher risk of incomplete tumor excision, potentially leading to recurrent disease and worse survival. NETs appear on macroscopic inspection as yellow-tan, firm nodules. Microscopic examination reveals submucosal conglomerates of cells organized in a nested or insular pattern.

The cytoplasm appears eosinophilic and finely granular, whereas the nuclei show the classic "salt-and-pepper" chromatin pattern. At immunohistochemistry characterization, tumors stain positive for synaptophysin and CgA, as well as for Ki-67, which is useful to determine the proliferative capacity of the lesion. The Ki-67 index is also a parameter assessed to stratify tumor grading. According to the World Health Organization grading systems, grade 1 is designated by a mitotic count of less than 2 per 2 mm^2 and Ki-67 less than or equal to 2%; grade 2 by a mitotic count between 2 and 20 per 2 mm^2 or Ki-67 of 3–20%; and grade 3 by a mitotic count of more than 20 per 2 mm^2 or Ki-67 index greater than 20%. NETs of the appendix are mostly grade 1 or grade 2 (Ki-67 index less than 20%). In the case of tumor grade 3, a GCC should be ruled out. Tumors of grade 1 and grade 2 usually show an indolent clinical course, with only a minority of them evolving into disseminated disease.

GCCs are rare appendiceal malignancies that exhibit a unique histological and biological profile, combining features of both adenocarcinomas and NETs. These tumors are composed of cells with partial neuroendocrine differentiation, which are intermixed with dysplastic signet-ring cells, leading to their distinct histopathological appearance.

Macroscopically, GCC often present as irregularly shaped lesions, lacking the well-defined borders typically seen in other appendiceal tumors. Their growth pattern is characterized by a predominant submucosal development, frequently displaying concentric infiltration of the appendiceal wall. Unlike conventional adenocarcinomas, GCCs tend to spare the mucosal layer, making early detection challenging. The tumor's growth may extend into the muscularis propria and beyond, sometimes invading adjacent structures, such as the periappendiceal fat or even nearby organs in advanced cases.

On microscopic examination, the neoplastic cells exhibit mild to intermediate degrees of atypia, with relatively low mitotic activity. This contributes to the tumor's often indolent appearance, though aggressive subtypes exist. The neoplastic goblet cells produce abundant intracytoplasmic mucin, which contributes to their resemblance to signet-ring cells seen in other malignancies, such as gastric or colorectal carcinomas.

Immunohistochemically, GCC display a characteristic staining pattern that aids in their differentiation from other appendiceal neoplasms. Neuroendocrine markers such as synaptophysin, chromogranin A (CgA), and CD56 are typically focally positive, reflecting the partial neuroendocrine differentiation of these tumors. Meanwhile, epithelial and mucin-associated markers, including cytokeratin 20 (CK20) and MUC2, show diffuse positivity, further distinguishing GCCs from pure NETs. This unique immunohistochemical profile plays a crucial role in accurate diagnosis, especially in cases where histopathological features overlap with other appendiceal malignancies.

Cases of primary lymphoma of the appendix have also been reported. NHL of B-cell origin is the most prevalent, with only a few cases of T-cell NHL described. Lymphocytes are normal dwellers of gastrointestinal tissues, so the differentiation between malignancy and physiologic reactive conditions is often problematic. The criteria for the diagnosis of primary tumors were provided to improve diagnostic yield, often employing a combination of immunohistochemistry and polymerase chain reaction analysis.

3.1.2 Diagnosis and follow-up

Neoplasms of the appendix are rarely suspected before surgical exploration and are most often discovered incidentally, either during an operation performed for unrelated conditions or on pathological examination of an appendectomy specimen. This delayed detection is largely due to the nonspecific and often subtle clinical presentation of these tumors.

Patients with appendiceal neoplasms may experience vague and insidious symptoms that are frequently overlooked or attributed to more common gastrointestinal disorders. These symptoms can include generalized fatigue, unintentional weight loss, chronic or intermittent abdominal pain, changes in bowel habits, and early satiety. In more advanced cases, the disease may manifest with signs of peritoneal involvement, including abdominal distension due to ascites, or systemic manifestations such as anemia and malaise. The insidious nature of these symptoms often leads to delayed diagnosis, allowing tumors to grow undetected until they reach a significant size or cause secondary complications.

In some cases, appendiceal tumors mimic acute appendicitis, presenting with right lower quadrant pain, fever, nausea, and vomiting. This overlap in symptomatology is particularly relevant for NETs and mucinous neoplasms, which can induce inflammation and luminal obstruction, leading to an appendicitis-like picture. Alternatively, larger neoplasms may exert a mass effect, particularly when they extend into the pelvis. This can result in compression of adjacent structures, leading to urinary symptoms such as dysuria, urinary frequency, or even ureteral obstruction with hydronephrosis. In women, compression of the reproductive organs may cause dyspareunia, menstrual irregularities, or nonspecific pelvic discomfort.

A thorough clinical assessment is crucial for identifying potential neoplastic processes. A detailed history should encompass prior surgical interventions, particularly previous appendectomies or abdominal procedures that might have included incidental appendiceal resections, as well as a review of symptoms suggestive of chronic or recurrent inflammation. The physical examination should include careful abdominal palpation to detect masses, tenderness, or signs of peritoneal irritation. A digital rectal examination is particularly valuable in evaluating pelvic involvement, as it can reveal large masses, assess mobility of surrounding structures, and detect the presence of peritoneal carcinomatosis through findings such as rectal nodularity or palpable ascitic fluid. In female patients, a bimanual pelvic examination may provide additional insights into the extent of disease spread.

In rare instances, mucinous tumors of the appendix can present in unusual ways, such as the detection of mucinous material within ventral, incisional, or inguinal hernias. This phenomenon, known as "pseudomyxoma hernia," occurs when gelatinous mucinous deposits extend into hernia sacs, often as a result of peritoneal dissemination. The presence of such mucinous deposits should raise suspicion for underlying appendiceal pathology, prompting further investigation through imaging and histopathological analysis.

Given the potential for appendiceal neoplasms to remain asymptomatic until advanced stages, maintaining a high index of suspicion is essential, particularly in patients with persistent or unexplained abdominal symptoms. A multimodal approach involving clinical assessment, imaging, and histopathology is necessary to achieve timely diagnosis and guide appropriate management strategies.

Patients with primary appendiceal neoplasms are at increased risk of synchronous colonic lesions, with a significant percentage of cases involving concurrent colorectal neoplasia. This association underscores the need for comprehensive gastrointestinal evaluation in individuals diagnosed with appendiceal tumors. The coexistence of colorectal neoplasms may be due to shared genetic or environmental risk factors, including underlying predispositions such as Lynch syndrome or familial adenomatous polyposis (FAP), both of which increase susceptibility to multiple gastrointestinal malignances.

Accurate preoperative diagnosis of epithelial appendiceal cancer is challenging due to the diverse clinical presentations and overlapping imaging characteristics of appendiceal neoplasms. Staging requires a complete CT scan of the thorax, abdomen, and pelvis. MRI is superior to CT in detecting mucin in the peritoneal cavity, utilizing diffusion-weighted imaging and delayed post-gadolinium sequences. MRI also helps predict the PCI before surgery and is useful in postoperative surveillance after cytoreductive surgery (CRS) and HIPEC. Preoperative suspicion of PMP is based on physical examination and imaging findings, with common features including abdominal distention and dullness to percussion. Imaging typically reveals ascites with secondary signs of extrinsic compression, such as scalloping of the liver or peritoneal reflection.

In theory, appendiceal tumors can be diagnosed via colonoscopy when they manifest as a protrusion, ulceration, or polypoid tissue at the appendiceal orifice. However, such findings are uncommon due to the retrocecal and intraperitoneal location of the appendix, which limits direct visualization. When a tumor infiltrates the cecum, colonoscopy may reveal mucosal abnormalities such as an extrinsic mass effect, mucosal irregularities, or focal thickening near the appendiceal opening. Despite these potential indicators, endoscopy has limited diagnostic value for appendiceal neoplasms, as small or isolated tumors are rarely visible through the colonic lumen. In cases of mucinous neoplasms, colonoscopy may occasionally detect mucoid extrusions from the appendiceal orifice, a finding suggestive of PMP.

Due to these limitations, imaging modalities play a more significant role in the detection and characterization of appendiceal neoplasms. Ultrasound, although commonly used in the initial assessment of right lower quadrant pain, is generally insufficient for definitive diagnosis. It may reveal nonspecific findings such as an appendiceal mass, focal wall thickening, or complex free fluid suggestive of peritoneal involvement. In some cases, mucinous tumors can present as cystic, hypoechoic structures with posterior acoustic enhancement, but these features are not pathognomonic.

Given these diagnostic challenges, cross-sectional imaging techniques such as computed tomography (CT) and magnetic resonance imaging (MRI) are more reliable for evaluating suspected appendiceal neoplasms. CT scanning, often performed for acute appendicitis or nonspecific abdominal symptoms, can incidentally reveal appendiceal masses, luminal dilatation, or associated peritoneal deposits. Contrast-enhanced CT is particularly useful in assessing tumor size, local invasion, and distant spread. MRI, especially with diffusion-weighted imaging, can further delineate mucinous tumors and detect subtle peritoneal dissemination.

Ultimately, while endoscopy and ultrasound have limited roles in diagnosing appendiceal neoplasms, they may provide indirect clues that prompt further investigation. A high degree of clinical suspicion, combined with advanced imaging techniques, is essential for early identification and appropriate management of these rare but significant malignancies.

While there are no studies specifically focusing on the diagnosis of appendiceal neuroendocrine cancer, the diagnostic approach aligns with that of small intestinal NETs. Preoperative evaluation should include a detailed history and physical examination, with attention to symptoms associated with carcinoid syndrome, such as facial flushing or profuse diarrhea. These systemic manifestations result from the secretion of hormones like growth hormone, gastrin, calcitonin, substance P, insulin, neurotensin, and serotonin. Due to first-pass hepatic metabolism, the effects of these hormones are rarely overt unless extensive liver metastases overpower this mechanism, leading to symptomatic disease. Laboratory studies play a crucial role in diagnosis, with chromogranin A (CgA) levels correlating with tumor burden. CgA is typically normal in tumors smaller than two centimeters but increases with larger tumors. Measurement of urinary 5-hydroxyindoleacetic acid (5-HIAA) is essential in cases of carcinoid syndrome. Although elevated levels of these biomarkers have been associated with poor prognosis, they are not reliable for diagnosing NETs or guiding treatment decisions.

NETs of the appendix primarily metastasize to the liver and lungs, following a predictable pattern of dissemination through hematogenous and lymphatic routes. Due to their potential for distant spread, accurate staging is essential for determining prognosis and guiding treatment decisions. This is best achieved through a combination of imaging modalities, including contrast-enhanced CT or MRI of the chest, abdomen, and pelvis.

Most appendiceal NETs express somatostatin receptors, making somatostatin receptor scintigraphy (SRS) a valuable tool for both initial staging and follow-up. SRS, using radiolabeled somatostatin analogs such as indium-111 pentetreotide or newer gallium-68–labeled agents, enables the detection of both primary and metastatic lesions. While modern CT and MRI provide excellent anatomical resolution, SRS remains particularly useful for confirming indeterminate findings, especially in patients with symptoms suggestive of carcinoid syndrome, such as flushing, diarrhea, and wheezing. The ability of SRS to identify small, functionally active metastases makes it an essential component of comprehensive staging.

Positron emission tomography (PET) combined with CT has emerged as another valuable tool for detecting metastatic neuroendocrine disease. PET-CT using gallium-68–labeled somatostatin analogs (such as Ga-68 DOTATATE) offers high sensitivity and specificity for identifying NET metastases, often outperforming conventional imaging techniques in detecting small or occult lesions. However, the routine use of PET-CT in appendiceal NET staging remains a topic of debate. While it provides superior lesion detection in select cases, its high cost and uncertain impact on treatment decisions necessitate careful patient selection. Current evidence suggests that PET imaging may aid in detecting metastatic disease but has not been shown to significantly improve staging accuracy or alter clinical management in most cases.

Ultimately, the optimal approach to staging appendiceal NETs involves a multimodal strategy tailored to the individual patient. Contrast-enhanced CT or MRI remains the cornerstone of initial staging, while SRS or PET-CT may be employed selectively for cases requiring further characterization of indeterminate lesions or for patients with suspected metastatic disease. The integration of these imaging modalities allows for a more precise assessment of tumor burden, facilitating appropriate therapeutic planning and long-term surveillance.

Surveillance for disease recurrence in patients with appendiceal NETs should be particularly rigorous in individuals who may be candidates for further treatment upon relapse. Given the potential for late recurrences, long-term follow-up is essential to detect disease progression at an early and potentially treatable stage.

Surveillance involves a combination of biochemical and radiographic assessments, with monitoring intervals typically ranging from 6 to 12 months based on tumor histologic grade, stage at diagnosis, and initial treatment response. Well-differentiated, low-grade NETs (G1) tend to have a more indolent course, allowing for less frequent follow-up, whereas high-grade (G3) or metastatic disease warrants more intensive surveillance. Despite the absence of universally standardized guidelines – largely due to the rarity of appendiceal NETs and their generally slow-growing nature – surveillance is commonly recommended for at least 10 years following curative resection. This extended duration accounts for the potential for late recurrences, particularly in cases with nodal involvement or incomplete initial staging.

Biochemical markers such as chromogranin A (CgA) and urinary or plasma 5-HIAA levels provide valuable insights into disease activity. Chromogranin A, a general marker of neuroendocrine differentiation, is commonly elevated in NETs and can serve as an indicator of tumor burden and response to therapy. Similarly, 5-HIAA, a serotonin metabolite, is particularly relevant in functional NETs, especially those associated with carcinoid syndrome. However, while these biomarkers can suggest disease recurrence, they lack specificity and must be interpreted in conjunction with imaging findings.

Radiographic surveillance remains the cornerstone of follow-up, with cross-sectional imaging modalities such as contrast-enhanced CT or MRI playing a primary role. These techniques allow for the detection of recurrent or metastatic disease, particularly in the liver, which is the most common site of distant spread. SRS, including gallium-68 DOTATATE PET-CT, is not routinely used for surveillance but may be employed in select cases where conventional imaging yields inconclusive findings. SRS can help confirm recurrence in patients with biochemical or clinical suspicion of disease progression, particularly if standard imaging fails to identify a lesion.

The choice of surveillance strategy should be individualized, taking into account tumor biology, patient comorbidities, and the potential for further therapeutic intervention. A structured follow-up protocol, integrating biomarker assessment and imaging at appropriate intervals, ensures timely detection of recurrence and facilitates early therapeutic decision-making, optimizing patient outcomes.

In the early stages, mucinous tumors of the appendix frequently mimic acute appendicitis, with right lower quadrant pain resulting from luminal distention by accumulating mucin. This overlap in presentation can lead to an initial misdiagnosis, with the true nature of the disease only becoming apparent upon pathological examination of an appendectomy specimen. However, unlike acute appendicitis, mucinous neoplasms often lack severe inflammatory findings, and the pain may be more chronic or intermittent rather than abrupt in onset. Even at advanced stages, intestinal obstruction is an uncommon primary manifestation, as mucinous tumors tend to spread within the peritoneal cavity rather than invade the bowel wall or cause extrinsic compression. Low-grade mucinous neoplasms often remain asymptomatic for years, with the slow accumulation of mucin gradually leading to increased abdominal girth, non-specific discomfort, and eventually pain due to mass effect. Conversely, high-grade disease tends to become clinically apparent at an earlier stage due to its aggressive biological behavior, which includes rapid tumor growth, invasion of adjacent structures, and a higher propensity for peritoneal dissemination. Once peritoneal spread occurs, the distribution of mucinous deposits follows the natural circulation of peritoneal fluid, preferentially accumulating in dependent areas such as the pelvis, paracolic gutters, and the omentum. Interestingly, peristaltic intestinal surfaces are frequently spared, a phenomenon attributed to the constant motion preventing mucin adherence. This characteristic pattern of spread influences both diagnostic imaging interpretation and surgical planning for cytoreduction.

Tumor markers play a significant role in the diagnosis, prognosis, and surveillance of appendiceal mucinous neoplasms. Carcinoembryonic antigen (CEA), carbohydrate antigen 19-9 (CA19-9), and cancer antigen 125 (CA-125) are routinely measured at initial diagnosis and throughout follow-up. In cases of mucinous adenocarcinoma, a normal baseline CA-125 level has been associated with a higher likelihood of achieving complete cytoreduction, highlighting its prognostic value. Conversely, elevated baseline CA19-9 has been linked to poorer survival and serves as a useful marker for detecting recurrence after CRS combined with HIPEC. Following complete cytoreduction, CEA levels typically normalize, while CA19-9 and CA-125 may remain elevated, reflecting persistent or recurrent disease. Notably, patients with normal preoperative tumor markers tend to experience significantly longer survival, suggesting that elevated markers may indicate a more aggressive tumor phenotype requiring perioperative systemic chemotherapy.

Surveillance strategies for disease recurrence integrate serial tumor marker evaluation with imaging studies. Cross-sectional imaging, particularly contrast-enhanced CT or MRI, is the primary modality for detecting peritoneal disease recurrence. In select cases, PET-CT or somatostatin receptor-based imaging may provide additional insights, particularly when standard imaging yields inconclusive results.

Recent advancements in molecular profiling have explored genetic alterations distinguishing low-grade from high-grade mucinous tumors. Key genetic markers under investigation include cyclooxygenase-2 (COX-2) expression and mutations in KRAS, TP53, and SMAD4. While these molecular characteristics hold promise for refining diagnostic classification and prognostication, their definitive impact on clinical management remains to be determined. As research progresses, molecular profiling may contribute to personalized therapeutic strategies, potentially guiding decisions on the need for systemic chemotherapy or targeted therapies.

3.1.3 Treatment

Appendiceal neoplasms are managed with a combination of surgery and, in select cases, chemotherapy, with the approach tailored to tumor histology, size, and disease stage. NETs of the appendix, which are often discovered incidentally during appendectomy, represent a unique subset of these neoplasms. Their management depends largely on tumor size, presence of adverse histologic features, and potential for metastatic spread.

For NETs confined to the appendix, tumor size is a key determinant of the surgical approach. Lesions measuring less than one centimeter, provided they lack unfavorable characteristics such as lymphovascular invasion, mesoappendiceal invasion, high mitotic rate, or an elevated Ki-67 proliferation index, are typically managed with a simple appendectomy. This procedure, which includes complete removal of the mesoappendix, is associated with excellent long-term survival, given the minimal risk of regional lymph node metastasis in these small tumors.

In contrast, tumors greater than two centimeters are considered to have a significantly higher risk of nodal involvement and distant spread. As a result, the standard surgical approach in such cases is a right hemicolectomy, which allows for a more extensive lymphadenectomy and resection of the ileocolic vascular supply to address potential microscopic disease. This procedure is necessary to improve oncologic outcomes and reduce recurrence risk.

For intermediate-sized NETs, measuring between one and two centimeters, surgical management is more nuanced. The decision to proceed with appendectomy alone versus right hemicolectomy is influenced by several additional histopathologic and clinical factors. Tumors demonstrating mesoappendiceal invasion, a high mitotic index, a Ki-67 index exceeding 3%, or evidence of lymphovascular invasion are at greater risk for regional spread, warranting a more aggressive surgical approach. Similarly, tumor location within the appendix plays a crucial role, as neoplasms situated at the base of the appendix may pose challenges for complete local excision and increase the likelihood of residual disease if an appendectomy is performed in isolation.

Beyond histologic and anatomic considerations, patient-specific factors such as age, comorbidities, and overall surgical risk must be taken into account when determining the optimal intervention. In pediatric patients, appendiceal NETs tend to have a more favorable prognosis, even when lesions exceed one centimeter in size. Studies have shown that, in children and adolescents, the rate of nodal metastasis remains low for small to intermediate-sized tumors, making appendectomy a reasonable approach in select cases where unfavorable features are absent. The management of appendiceal NETs requires a multidisciplinary approach, incorporating surgical expertise, histopathologic assessment, and, in some cases, additional oncologic evaluation to ensure optimal outcomes.

The management of adenocarcinomas of the appendix, particularly the choice between appendectomy and right hemicolectomy, remains a subject of debate among clinicians. This controversy stems from the varying biological behaviors and clinical outcomes associated with different subtypes of appendiceal tumors, such as LAMNs and HAMNs (high-grade appendiceal mucinous neoplasms).

LAMNs, which are characterized by their slow-growing and indolent nature, generally have a favorable prognosis. Studies have shown that appendectomy alone is often sufficient for treating LAMNs, especially in cases where there is no evidence of perforation or peritoneal involvement. In such scenarios, the recurrence rates after appendectomy are notably low, making it a viable and less invasive treatment option. However, the surgical approach must be carefully considered. If laparoscopic resection is deemed unsafe or technically challenging due to factors such as tumor size or location, conversion to an open procedure is recommended. This approach minimizes the risk of iatrogenic rupture during surgery, which could lead to the dissemination of mucin or tumor cells into the peritoneal cavity, potentially complicating the patient's prognosis.

For HAMNs, which are more aggressive than LAMNs but still confined to the appendix, appendectomy may also be adequate, provided that thorough pathological examination excludes the presence of invasive adenocarcinoma. Invasive adenocarcinoma would necessitate more extensive surgical intervention, such as right hemicolectomy, due to the higher risk of lymph node involvement and distant metastasis.

An important consideration in the treatment of non-perforated LAMNs is the status of the resection margin. Even if the resection margin is microscopically positive after appendectomy, this finding does not always correlate with an increased risk of recurrence or the need for additional surgery, such as right hemicolectomy. This highlights the importance of individualized treatment planning, taking into account the specific histopathological features of the tumor, the patient's overall health, and the potential risks and benefits of further surgical intervention.

Appendiceal adenocarcinoma spreads to regional lymph nodes at varying rates, with higher nodal involvement in non-mucinous variants. Therefore, right hemicolectomy is generally recommended for non-mucinous adenocarcinoma confined to the appendix, as it allows for comprehensive staging and potential therapeutic benefit. Interestingly, LAMNs exhibit a greater tendency for peritoneal metastasis but a lower incidence of lymph node involvement compared to HAMNs. Right colectomy is also advised for appendiceal goblet cell adenocarcinoma due to its aggressive nature. Patients with goblet cell adenocarcinoma and peritoneal metastases may be candidates for CRS and intraoperative chemotherapy, with complete cytoreduction achievable in many cases.

While some advocate for right hemicolectomy in all adenocarcinomas for radicality and staging, efforts have been made to stratify patients by risk of lymph node metastasis. Studies suggest that only HAMNs and non-mucinous adenocarcinomas should undergo right colon resection, leading to the concept of radical appendectomy. Interval right hemicolectomy is recommended when radical appendectomy reveals mesoappendiceal lymph node metastases. Radical appendectomy involves en bloc removal of the appendix, surrounding tissues, and lymph nodes, with the appendiceal artery ligated at its origin. If nodal metastases are detected, formal right colectomy is performed. Non-mucinous adenocarcinomas require immediate right colon resection due to high nodal positivity rates.

Routine right hemicolectomy is not advised in patients with overt peritoneal metastases. Historically, treatment involved repeated mucinous ascites drainage and tumor debulking. However, studies have not demonstrated a survival advantage of right colectomy over appendectomy alone in patients undergoing CRS and HIPEC. Nodal positivity without peritoneal spread is associated with poor prognosis despite extensive resection. Nonetheless, right colectomy may be necessary for complete cytoreduction in cases of extensive peritoneal disease.

HIPEC delivers high intraperitoneal doses of heated chemotherapy with minimal systemic toxicity. CRS and HIPEC are most effective in low PCI scores, low-grade tumors, and complete cytoreduction. Hyperthermia exerts cytotoxic effects on malignant cells and enhances chemotherapeutic efficacy. CRS aims to eradicate visible disease before HIPEC administration. It includes selective peritonectomies, excision of tumor implants, supracolic omentectomy, and resection of affected organs. Postoperative morbidity varies widely, though long-term survivors report improved quality of life.

Patient selection is essential for treatment planning. Preoperative imaging determines the extent of resectable disease, and diagnostic laparoscopy can estimate cytoreduction feasibility. Peritoneal disease is assessed using the PCI or the Peritoneal Surface Disease Severity Score. Successful cytoreduction is expected in patients without biliary, ureteral, or bowel obstruction. Women should be counseled on bilateral salpingo-oophorectomy due to the risk of occult ovarian metastases. Limited peritoneal involvement by acellular mucin in LAMNs may be managed with appendectomy and regional cytoreduction, whereas cellular mucin necessitates HIPEC.

Following CRS, intraperitoneal chemotherapy should be administered. HIPEC reduces recurrence and improves survival compared to debulking surgery alone. Systemic chemotherapy, including bevacizumab, has shown benefits in unresectable cases. Preoperative chemotherapy allows for disease response assessment and patient tolerance evaluation. Other intraoperative chemotherapy methods, such as early postoperative intraperitoneal chemotherapy, provide comparable outcomes. However, targeted therapies based on cyclooxygenase-2 expression and KRAS mutations have not improved survival.

Primary appendiceal lymphomas are relatively uncommon and are typically managed with an appendectomy, which may be curative in cases where the disease is confined to the appendix. However, depending on the histological subtype, tumor size, and presence of high-risk features, adjuvant chemotherapy or radiotherapy may be considered to reduce the risk of recurrence. In cases where the lymphoma has invaded the mesoappendix or has spread to regional lymph nodes, a more extensive surgical approach, such as ileocecal resection, is warranted to ensure complete removal of the disease. When the lymphoma is more widespread or involves adjacent structures, a right hemicolectomy is the preferred surgical option to achieve adequate oncologic control.

3.2 Secondary malignancies

3.2.1 Introduction

Secondary malignancies of the appendix are rare clinical entities, often discovered incidentally during surgical procedures or imaging studies performed for other indications. Unlike primary appendiceal tumors, which include epithelial neoplasms, carcinoid tumors, and lymphomas, secondary malignancies arise from metastatic spread of cancers originating in distant organs. The appendix is generally considered an uncommon site for metastasis due to its small size, narrow lumen, and limited blood supply; however, when metastases do occur, they are most frequently associated with primary tumors of the gastrointestinal tract, gynecological malignancies, or hematologic cancers.

The clinical presentation of secondary appendiceal malignancies is often nonspecific, with symptoms ranging from asymptomatic incidental findings to acute appendicitis, bowel obstruction, or perforation. This diagnostic challenge underscores the importance of histopathological evaluation in cases where atypical appendiceal pathology is suspected. Imaging studies, such as CT and PET, may aid in detecting appendiceal involvement in patients with known metastatic disease.

Given the rarity of secondary malignancies in the appendix, standardized treatment protocols are lacking. Management depends on factors such as the primary tumor type, extent of metastatic disease, and overall patient prognosis. In some cases, appendectomy alone may be sufficient for localized involvement, while more extensive surgical resection is warranted if the appendix is part of a widespread metastatic process. Systemic therapy remains the cornerstone of treatment for most cases, particularly when appendiceal involvement is part of disseminated malignancy.

This chapter explores the epidemiology, pathogenesis, clinical manifestations, diagnostic approaches, and therapeutic strategies for secondary malignancies of the appendix, providing insights into this uncommon but clinically significant condition.

3.2.2 Epidemiology and pathogenesis

Epidemiological data on metastatic involvement of the appendix are limited, as most published cases exist within case reports or small case series. However, studies suggest that the incidence of secondary appendiceal malignancies is significantly lower than that of primary tumors, accounting for a small fraction of all appendiceal neoplasms. The most common primary sources of metastatic disease to the appendix include gastrointestinal malignancies – particularly colorectal, gastric, and pancreatic cancers – gynecological tumors such as ovarian and endometrial carcinomas, and hematologic malignancies, especially NHLand leukemias. Other reported sources include breast cancer, lung cancer, melanoma, and genitourinary malignancies, although these are considerably rarer. The increased frequency of appendiceal metastases from ovarian and gastrointestinal cancers is likely due to their propensity for peritoneal dissemination, which can involve the appendix through direct implantation.

The pathogenesis of secondary malignancies in the appendix depends largely on the mode of metastatic spread, which may occur via direct extension, hematogenous dissemination, lymphatic spread, or peritoneal seeding. Direct invasion from adjacent tumors, such as cecal or ovarian cancers, is a relatively common mechanism, given the anatomical proximity of the appendix to these structures. Peritoneal carcinomatosis, often seen in advanced-stage gastrointestinal and gynecological malignancies, can also lead to secondary involvement of the appendix through transcoelomic spread, where malignant cells implant onto the serosal surface and subsequently invade deeper layers of the appendiceal wall. This pattern of dissemination is frequently observed in mucinous neoplasms, such as PMP originating from appendiceal or ovarian tumors, which can engulf the appendix in a gelatinous accumulation of malignant mucin-producing cells. Hematogenous and lymphatic spread, while less common, may be observed in metastatic involvement from distant organs, including breast and lung carcinomas, as well as in hematologic malignancies such as leukemias and lymphomas, where malignant cells infiltrate the appendiceal wall via the bloodstream or lymphatic channels.

Despite these various mechanisms, the appendix remains an infrequent site of metastasis, likely due to its anatomical and physiological characteristics. Its small caliber, limited direct vascular supply, and relatively isolated location within the peritoneal cavity may reduce the likelihood of tumor implantation or direct invasion. Furthermore, the immune activity within the appendiceal-associated lymphoid tissue could play a protective role in preventing metastatic colonization.

3.2.3 Diagnostic approaches and treatment strategies

The diagnosis and management of secondary malignancies of the appendix require a comprehensive, individualized approach due to their rarity and often incidental discovery. Unlike primary appendiceal neoplasms, which may present with specific clinical syndromes such as PMP or neuroendocrine tumor-related symptoms, secondary malignancies are frequently asymptomatic or mimic acute appendicitis, making preoperative diagnosis challenging. Imaging techniques such as CT, MRI, and PET scans play a crucial role in identifying appendiceal involvement, particularly in patients with a known primary malignancy. CT is often the first-line modality and can reveal subtle abnormalities such as appendiceal wall thickening, luminal distension, or an associated mass, while MRI is useful for characterizing peritoneal involvement, especially in mucinous tumors. PET scans may help detect hypermetabolic appendiceal lesions in cases of metastatic spread from solid tumors or hematologic malignancies, though their sensitivity can be variable depending on the metabolic activity of the tumor. Despite advances in imaging, definitive diagnosis relies on histopathological examination following appendectomy, biopsy, or more extensive surgical resection. In cases where secondary malignancies arise from direct invasion, such as from cecal adenocarcinoma or ovarian carcinoma, colonoscopy may provide additional diagnostic clues, including extrinsic compression of the appendiceal orifice or mucosal abnormalities suggestive of contiguous spread. However, peritoneal seeding or hematogenous dissemination may not be readily identifiable through endoscopic evaluation, necessitating laparoscopic exploration in select cases where suspicion remains high.

Once a secondary appendiceal malignancy is diagnosed, treatment must be tailored to the patient's overall oncologic status, the extent of disease, and the nature of the primary malignancy. In cases where the appendix is an isolated site of metastasis and the underlying cancer is well-controlled, an appendectomy alone may suffice, particularly if the lesion is detected incidentally and has not compromised adjacent structures. However, more extensive surgical intervention is often required when the appendix is involved in widespread metastatic disease. If the malignancy has spread to the mesoappendix or regional lymph nodes, a right hemicolectomy may be indicated to achieve complete oncologic resection and prevent disease progression. This approach is particularly relevant when the appendix is affected by direct invasion from a cecal tumor, as the risk of local recurrence or incomplete resection is higher with a limited surgical approach. CRS with HIPEC is often employed in cases of peritoneal carcinomatosis, particularly in appendiceal mucinous neoplasms or ovarian cancers, where complete cytoreduction is associated with improved long-term survival. For patients with hematologic malignancies such as NHL or leukemia, surgical resection may play a more limited role, as systemic therapy is the primary treatment modality. Chemotherapy remains a cornerstone of management for most secondary appendiceal malignancies, with regimens tailored to the underlying primary tumor. Fluoropyrimidine-based chemotherapy, such as FOLFOX or FOLFIRI, is commonly used in colorectal cancer metastases, while platinum-based regimens like carboplatin and paclitaxel are preferred for ovarian cancer. Targeted therapies, including EGFR inhibitors in colorectal cancer, PARP inhibitors in BRCA-mutated ovarian cancer, and tyrosine kinase inhibitors in GISTs, have expanded treatment options and may improve outcomes in select cases. Immunotherapy with checkpoint inhibitors is increasingly being explored for microsatellite instability-high tumors and hematologic malignancies with actionable mutations.

While radiotherapy is rarely utilized in the treatment of secondary appendiceal malignancies, it may be considered in specific scenarios, such as localized lymphomatous involvement of the appendix or for palliative purposes in advanced metastatic disease. In patients with extensive metastases and limited treatment options, palliative care becomes a critical component of management, focusing on symptom relief and quality of life. Interventions such as percutaneous drainage of malignant ascites, endoscopic stenting for bowel obstruction, and analgesic regimens tailored to cancer-related pain can significantly improve patient comfort. Given the complexity of secondary appendiceal malignancies, a multidisciplinary approach involving surgical oncologists, medical oncologists, radiologists, and pathologists is essential to ensure optimal diagnostic and therapeutic strategies. Ongoing research into molecular profiling and personalized medicine may further refine treatment approaches, offering improved prognostic insights and more effective therapeutic options for patients with metastatic disease involving the appendix.

References

- Smeenk RM, Verwaal VVM. Appendiceal neoplasms and pseudomyxoma peritonei: A population based study. Eur J Surg Oncol. 2008; 34: 196–201.
- Smeenk RM, Verwaal VVM, Zoetmulder VJ. Appendiceal neoplasms and pseudomyxoma peritonei: a population based study. Eur J Surg Oncol. 2008; 34: 196–201.
- Dm MJAS. Carcinoid tumors of the appendix: a population-based study. J Surg Oncol. 2011; 104: 41–44.
- Scott A, Upadhyay V. Carcinoid tumours of the appendix in children in Auckland, New Zealand. NZ Med J. 2011; 124: 56–60.
- Carcinoids (argentaffin-cell tumors) and nerve hyperplasia of the appendicular mucosa. Am J Pathol. 1928; 4: 181–212.
- Giacinto D, Rizza RF. Chromogranin a: from laboratory to clinical aspects of patients with neuroendocrine tumors. Int J Endocrinol. 2018.
- Alexandraki KI, Bramis GJ, Ballian KI, Dimitriou N, Giannakakis N, Tsigris T, et al. Clinical value of right hemicolectomy for appendiceal carcinoids using pathologic criteria. J Endocrinol Invest. 2011; 34: 255–59.
- Davison JM, Pingpank CH. Clinicopathologic and molecular analysis of disseminated appendiceal mucinous neoplasms: identification of factors predicting survival and proposed criteria for a three-tiered assessment of tumor grade. Mod Pathol. 2014; 27: 1521–39.
- Gupta S, Adsay PV. Clinicopathological analysis of primary epithelial appendiceal neoplasms. Med Oncol. 2010; 27: 1073–78.
- Jiang Y, Wang LH, Liu W, Tang H, Zhang Y. Clinicopathological features and immunoexpression profiles of goblet cell carcinoid and typical carcinoid of the appendix. Pathol Oncol Res. 2011; 17: 127–32.
- Singh S, Chan ML. Commonwealth Neuroendocrine Tumour Collaboration (CommNETS) Follow-up Working Group. Follow-up recommendations for completely resected gastroenteropancreatic neuroendocrine tumors. JAMA Oncol. 2018; 4: 1597–604.
- Goldstein D, Ej WK. Comprehensive genomic profiling of cancer of the appendix to reveal new routes to targeted therapies. J Clin Oncol. 2015; 33: 606–608.
- Otoole D, Gross GA, Delle Fave D, Barkmanova G, Connor O, Pape J, et al. Consensus Conference and European Neuroendocrine Tumors: ENETS Consensus Guidelines for the Standards of Care in Neuroendocrine Tumors: biochemical markers. Neuroendocrinology. 2009; 90: 194–202.
- Oberg K, De Herder MI. Consensus on biomarkers for neuroendocrine tumour disease. Lancet Oncol. 2015; 16: e435–46.
- Ji H, Seidman IC. Cytokeratins 7 and 20, Dpc4, and MUC5AC in the distinction of metastatic mucinous carcinomas in the ovary from primary ovarian mucinous tumors: Dpc4 assists in identifying metastatic pancreatic carcinomas. Int J Gynecol Pathol. 2002; 21: 391–400.
- Gouffon M, Ziegler IS. Diagnosis and workup of 522 consecutive patients with neuroendocrine neoplasms in Switzerland. Swiss Med Wkly. 2014; 144.
- Pape UF, Costa NB, Gross F, Kelestimur D, Kianmanesh F, Knigge R, et al. ENETS consensus guidelines for neuroendocrine neoplasms of the appendix (excluding goblet cell carcinomas). Neuroendocrinology. 2016; 103: 144–52.
- Chetty R. Gastro-intestinal Kaposi's sarcoma, with special reference to the appendix. S Afr J Surg. 1999; 37: 9–11.
- Burke AP, Federspiel SL, Shekitka BH, Helwig KM. Goblet cell carcinoids and related tumors of the vermiform appendix. Am J Clin Pathol. 1990; 94: 27–35.
- Turaga KK, Gamblin PS. Importance of histologic subtype in the staging of appendiceal tumors. Ann Surg Oncol. 2012; 19: 1379–85.

- Overman MJ, Hu FK. Improving the AJCC/TNM staging for adenocarcinomas of the appendix: the prognostic impact of histological grade. Ann Surg. 2013; 257: 1072–78.
- Shaibwl GM, Chen Z. Incidence and survival of appendiceal mucinous neoplasms: A SEER analysis. Am J Clin Oncol. 2017; 40: 569–73.
- Lohsiriwat V, Lohsiriwat VA. Incidence of synchronous appendiceal neoplasm in patients with colorectal cancer and its clinical significance. World J Surg Oncol. 2009; 7.
- Mcgory ML, Kang MM. Malignancies of the appendix: beyond case series reports. Dis Colon Rectum. 2005; 48: 2264–71.
- Kj K. Management of Appendix Cancer. Clin Colon Rectal Surg. 2015; 28: 247–55.
- Szych C, Connolly SA. Molecular genetic evidence supporting the clonality and appendiceal origin of pseudomyxoma peritonei in women. Am J Pathol. 1999; 154: 1849–55.
- Khatti S, Medeiros FS, Szklaruk LJ. Myeloid sarcoma of the appendix mimicking acute appendicitis. AJR Am J Roentgenol. 2004; 182: 247.
- Damore F, Grønbæk BH, Thorling K, Pedersen K, Jensen M. Non-Hodgkin's lymphoma of the gastrointestinal tract: a population-based analysis of incidence, geographic distribution, clinicopathologic presentation features, and prognosis. J Clin Oncol. 1994; 12: 1673–84.
- Yao JC, Phan HM. One hundred years after 'carcinoid': epidemiology of and prognostic factors for neuroendocrine tumors in 35,825 cases in the United States. J Clin Oncol. 2008; 26: 3063–72.
- Bolanowski M, Bobek-Billewicz BT. Polish network of neuroendocrine tumours. neuroendocrine neoplasms of the small intestine and the appendix: management guidelines (recommended by the polish network of neuroendocrine tumours). Endokrynol Pol. 2013; 64: 480–93.
- Ozakyol AH, Kabukcuoglu ST. Primary appendiceal adenocarcinoma. Am J Clin Oncol. 1999; 22: 458–59.
- Aw E. Primary carcinoma of the vermiform appendix, with a report of three cases. Ann Surg. 1903; 37: 549–74.
- Mori M, Kikunoki KT, Motoori M, Sugimachi T. Primary malignant lymphoma of the appendix. Jpn J Surg. 1985; 15: 230–33.
- Mccusker ME, Clegg CT. Primary malignant neoplasms of the appendix: A population based study from the surveillance, epidemiology and end-results program, 1973–1998. Cancer. 1973; 94: 3307–12.
- Kitamura Y, Terada OT. Primary T-cell non-Hodgkin's malignant lymphoma of the appendix. Pathol Int. 2000; 50: 313–17.
- Levine EA, Qasem VK, Philip SA, Cummins J, Chou KA, Ruiz JW, et al. Prognostic molecular subtypes of lowgrade cancer of the appendix. J Am Coll Surg. 2016; 222: 493–503.
- Rh Y. Pseudomyxoma peritonei and selected other aspects of the spread of appendiceal neoplasms. Semin Diagn Pathol. 2004; 21: 134–50.
- Bradley RF, Russell SJT. Pseudomyxoma peritonei of appendiceal origin: A clinicopathologic analysis of 101 patients uniformly treated at a single institution, with literature review. Am J Surg Pathol. 2006; 30: 551–59.
- Sm KJAH. Recent updates on neuroendocrine tumors from the gastrointestinal and pancreatobiliary tracts. Arch Pathol Lab Med. 2016; 140: 437–48.
- Dawson I, Morson CJ. Report of 37 cases with a study of factors influencing prognosis. Br J Surg. 1961; 49: 80–89.
- Deppen SA, Blume LE. Safety and efficacy of 68Ga-DOTATATE PET/CT for diagnosis, staging, and treatment management of neuroendocrine tumors. J Nucl Med. 2016; 57: 708–14.
- Pham TH, Abraham WB, Drelichman SC. Surgical and chemotherapy treatment outcomes of goblet cell carcinoid: a tertiary cancer center experience. Ann Surg Oncol. 2006; 13: 370–76.
- Dc C. The genetic basis of colorectal cancer: Insights into critical pathways of tumorigenesis. Gastroenterology. 2000; 119: 854–65.

- Van Den Heuvel MG, Verhoeven LV. The incidence of mucinous appendiceal malignancies: A population-based study. Int J Colorectal Dis. 2013; 28: 1307–10.
- Marmor S, Tuttle PP, Virnig TM. The rise in appendiceal cancer incidence: 2000–2009. J Gastrointest Surg. 2015; 19: 743–50.
- Munoz-Zuluaga CA, Macdonald SA. The role of preoperative tumor markers in patients with peritoneal carcinomatosis from appendiceal cancer undergoing cytoreductive surgery and hyperthermic intraperitoneal chemotherapy. Ann Surg Oncol. 2018; 25: 155–6.
- Rindi G, Couvelard KG. TNM staging of midgut and hindgut (neuro)endocrine tumors: a consensus proposal including a grading system. Virchows Arch. 2007; 451: 757–62.
- KE H, Hatch BD, Wertheimer-Hatch GF, Davis L, Foster GB. Tumors of the appendix and colon. World J Surg. 2000; 24: 430–36.
- Rohani P, Shen SS. Use of FDG-PET imaging for patients with disseminated cancer of the appendix. Am Surg. 2010; 76: 1338–44.
- Organization WH. WHO Classification of Tumours of the Digestive System. Lyon, France: IARC Press, 2010.

Index

https://doi.org/10.1515/9783112219782-004